Practical Case Studies in Hypertension Management

Series Editor
Giuliano Tocci
Rome, Italy

The aim of the book series "Practical Case Studies in Hypertension Management" is to provide physicians who treat hypertensive patients having different cardiovascular risk profiles with an easy-to-access tool that will enhance their clinical practice, improve average blood pressure control, and reduce the incidence of major hypertension-related complications. To achieve these ambitious goals, each volume presents and discusses a set of paradigmatic clinical cases relating to different scenarios in hypertension. These cases will serve as a basis for analyzing best practice and highlight problems in implementing the recommendations contained in international guidelines regarding diagnosis and treatment. While the available guidelines have contributed significantly in improving the diagnostic process, cardiovascular risk stratification, and therapeutic management in patients with essential hypertension, they are of limited help to physicians in daily clinical practice when approaching individual patients with hypertension, and this is particularly true when choosing among different drug classes and molecules. By discussing exemplary clinical cases that may better represent clinical practice in a "real world" setting, this series will assist physicians in selecting the best diagnostic and therapeutic options.

More information about this series at http://www.springer.com/series/13624

Raffaele Izzo

Hypertension and Cardiac Organ Damage

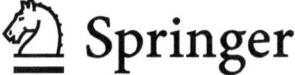 Springer

Raffaele Izzo
Hypertension Research Center (CIRIAPA)
University of Naples Federico II
Naples
Italy

ISSN 2364-6632   ISSN 2364-6640   (electronic)
Practical Case Studies in Hypertension Management
ISBN 978-3-319-56079-3   ISBN 978-3-319-56080-9   (eBook)
DOI 10.1007/978-3-319-56080-9

Library of Congress Control Number: 2017940405

Printed on acid-free paper

This Springer imprint is published by Springer Nature
The registered company is Springer International Publishing AG
The registered company address is: Gewerbestrasse 11, 6330 Cham, Switzerland

Foreword

Essential hypertension is a major contributor for developing cardiac abnormalities and diseases, such as left ventricular remodelling and/or hypertrophy, coronary artery disease, myocardial infarction, and congestive heart failure. In addition, several clinical studies demonstrated that hypertensive patients frequently showed other non-conventional cardiac abnormalities, mostly including left atrial enlargement, atrial fibrillation, sclerosis and dilatation of the aortic bulbus, and systolic and/or diastolic dysfunction. Although not included among markers of cardiac organ damage by current international guidelines, all these conditions lead to an increased risk of major cardiovascular and cerebrovascular outcomes. Indeed, it should be also noted that, beyond the established clinical conditions (i.e. coronary artery disease, previous myocardial infarction, and congestive heart failure), all these functional and structural abnormalities at the heart level can be treated with specific drug classes of antihypertensive agents, which have proven to delay progression and promote regression of such alterations. For these reasons, early identification and prompt treatment of cardiac organ damage is mandatory in all hypertensive patients, in order to achieve effective prevention of hypertension-related complications. In addition, the presence of these markers of organ damage can be used not only to identify high-risk hypertensive patients but also to monitor the effectiveness of a given antihypertensive regimen, beyond the blood pressure reductions.

In this volume of *Practical Case Studies in Hypertension Management*, the clinical management of paradigmatic cases of patients with hypertension and cardiac organ damage will be discussed, focusing on the different diagnostic criteria currently available for identifying early or advanced cardiac impairment or dysfunction, as well as on the different therapeutic options currently recommended for achieving effective and sustained blood pressure control and reducing hypertension-related morbidity and mortality in this high-risk populations.

Rome, Italy   Giuliano Tocci

Acknowledgement

I thank Dr Maria Virginia Manzi for her valuable contribution.

Contents

xvi   Contents

Clinical Case 1
Patient with Hypertension and Left Atrial Enlargement

1.1 Clinical Case Presentation

A 71-year-old Caucasian male was admitted to the outpatient clinic for hypertension and palpitations. He referred history of essential hypertension persisting for more than 4 years, treated with nifedipine GITS 30 mg once a day. The average values of home blood pressure were 130/80 mmHg.

Family History

Both parents and one brother (47 years old) have history of arterial hypertension.

Clinical History

Former smoker (about 10–20 cigarettes daily) for more than 30 years until the age of 55, he does not present additional cardiovascular risk factors, associated clinical conditions or non-cardiovascular diseases.

R. Izzo, *Hypertension and Cardiac Organ Damage*,
Practical Case Studies in Hypertension Management,
DOI 10.1007/978-3-319-56080-9_1,
© Springer International Publishing AG 2017

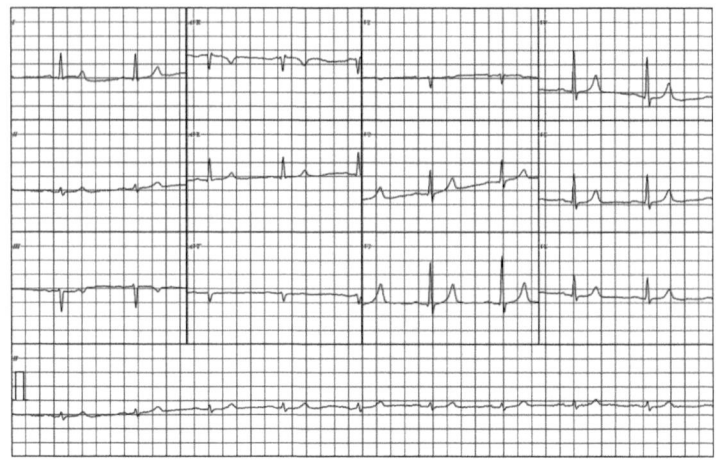

FIGURE 1.1 Electrocardiogram at the first available visit

Physical Examination

- Weight: 79 kg
- Height: 160 cm
- Body mass index (BMI): 30.8 kg/m^2
- Waist circumference: 108 cm
- Respiration: normal
- Heart exam: S1–S2 regular, normal and no murmurs
- Resting pulse: regular rhythm with normal heart rate (60 beats/min) (Fig. 1.1)
- Carotid arteries: no murmurs
- Femoral and foot arteries: palpable

Haematological Profile

- Haemoglobin: 14.5 g/dL
- Haematocrit: 45%
- Fasting plasma glucose: 102 mg/dL
- Lipid profile: total cholesterol (TOT-C), 131 mg/dL; low-density lipoprotein cholesterol (LDL-C), 70 mg/dL; high-density lipoprotein cholesterol (HDL-C), 39 mg/dL; triglycerides (TG), 110 mg/dL

- Electrolytes: sodium, 144 mEq/L; potassium, 4.2 mEq/L
- Serum uric acid: 5.9 mg/dL
- Renal function: urea, 39 mg/dL; creatinine, 0.9 mg/dL; creatinine clearance (Cockroft-Gault), 84.6 mL/min; estimated glomerular filtration rate (eGFR) (MDRD), 99 mL/min/1.73 m^2
- Urine analysis (dipstick): normal
- Albuminuria: 11.9 mg/24 h
- Liver function tests: normal
- Thyroid function tests: normal

Blood Pressure Profile

- Home BP (average): 125/75 mmHg
- Sitting BP: 130/85 mmHg (right arm); 130/80 mmHg (left arm)
- Standing BP: 125/85 mmHg at 1 min

12-Lead Electrocardiogram

Sinus rhythm with normal heart rate (57 bpm), normal atrio-ventricular and intraventricular conduction and normal ST segment without signs of LVH (Fig. 1.1).

Vascular Ultrasound

Both common carotids present an increase of the intima-media thickness (right, 1.3 mm, left, 1.0 mm) without evidence of significant atherosclerotic plaques.

Echocardiogram

Eccentric LV hypertrophy (LV mass indexed 56.2 g/m$^{2.7}$, relative wall thickness 0.33) with normal chamber dimension (LV end-diastolic diameter 54 mm), impaired LV relaxation (E/A ratio = 0.71), normal ejection fraction (LV ejection fraction 62%).

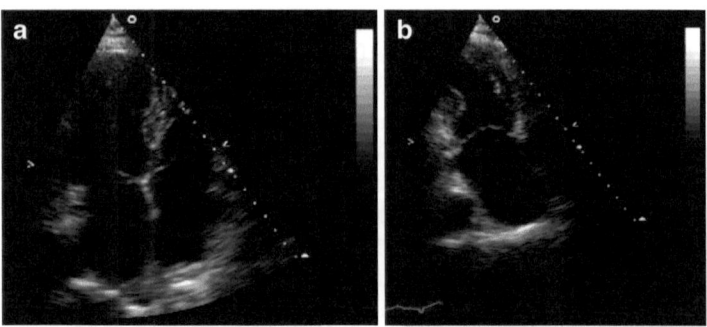

FIGURE 1.2 Echocardiogram at the first available visit (Panel a: 4 chamber; panel b: 2 chamber)

Normal dimension of aortic root and left atrial dilatation (49.45 cm^3/m^2). Right ventricle with normal dimension and function. Pericardium without relevant abnormalities (Fig. 1.2).

Mitral (+) and aortic (+) regurgitations at Doppler ultrasound examination.

Current Treatment

Nifedipine GITS 30 mg once a day.

Diagnosis

Essential hypertension with satisfactory BP control. Cardiac organ damage (concentric LV hypertrophy) and impaired LV relaxation. Additional cardiovascular risk factors (visceral obesity).

Q1: Which is the global cardiovascular risk profile in this patient?

1. Low
2. Moderate
3. High
4. Very high

Global Cardiovascular Risk Stratification

Echocardiography reveals signs of cardiac organ damage (eccentric LV hypertrophy) which, per se, is able to modify the individual global cardiovascular risk profile. On the basis of the echocardiographic assessment, this patient presents a high cardiovascular risk profile, according to the 2013 European Society of Hypertension (ESH)/European Society of Cardiology (ESC) global cardiovascular risk stratification [1].

Treatment Evaluation

- Stop nifedipine
- Start telmisartan 80 mg once a day

Prescriptions

- Periodical BP evaluation at home according to recommendations from guidelines
- Regular physical activity and low caloric intake
- ECG Holter monitoring

1.2   Follow-Up (Visit 1) at 6 Weeks

At follow-up visit, the patient is still symptomatic for dyspnoea. He now practices moderate physical activity two times per week with beneficial effects (weight loss). He also reports good adherence to prescribed medications without adverse reactions or drug-related side effects, but still has palpitations.

Physical Examination

- Weight: 76 kg
- Resting pulse: irregular rhythm with normal heart rate, 68 beats/min

- Respiration: signs of fluid overload in the lower lung field
- Heart sounds: S1–S2 regular, normal and no murmurs

Blood Pressure Profile

- Home BP (average): 120/75 mmHg
- Sitting BP: 125/85 mmHg
- Standing BP: 130/80 mmHg

Current Treatment

- Telmisartan 80 mg/die

12-Lead Electrocardiogram

Atrial fibrillation with average heart rate 79 bpm (Fig. 1.3).

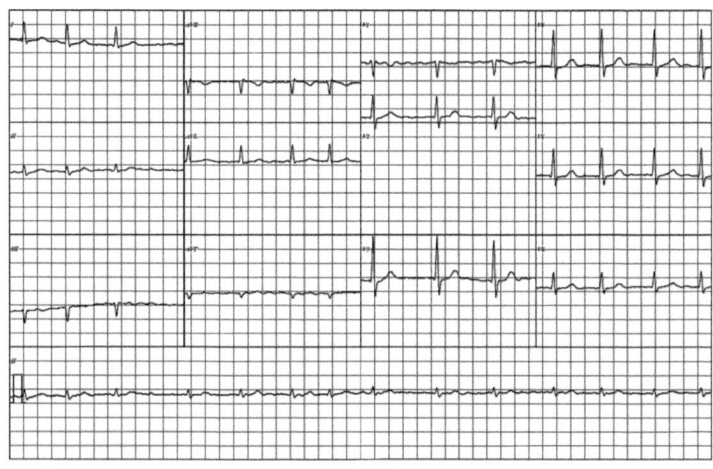

FIGURE 1.3 12-lead electrocardiogram at follow-up visit 1

ECG Holter Monitoring

Atrial fibrillation during all monitoring period. Mean heart rate 79 bpm (range 44–110). No ventricular arrhythmias. Maximum R–R 2234 ms.

Diagnosis

Atrial fibrillation in patient with essential hypertension with satisfactory BP control. Cardiac organ damage (concentric LV hypertrophy). Additional cardiovascular risk factors (visceral obesity).

> **Q2: Which is the best therapeutic option in this patient?**
> Possible answers are:
>
> 1. Add another antihypertensive drug.
> 2. Switch from angiotensin receptor blocker to beta-blocker.
> 3. Add an antiplatelet.
> 4. Add a NOAC (new oral anticoagulant) + a diuretic.

Prescriptions

- Telmisartan 80 mg (confirmed).
- Start rivaroxaban 20 mg once a day.
- Start torasemide 10 mg once a day.

1.3   Follow-Up (Visit 2) at 10 Weeks

At follow-up visit, the patient is asymptomatic for dyspnoea. He continues to practice moderate physical activity two times per week with beneficial effects. He also reports good adherence to prescribed medications without adverse reactions or drug-related side effects.

Physical Examination

- Weight: 75 kg
- Resting pulse: irregular rhythm with normal heart rate, 67 beats/min
- Respiration: normal
- Heart sounds: S1–S2 regular, normal and no murmurs

Blood Pressure Profile

- Home BP (average): 120/75 mmHg
- Sitting BP: 125/80 mmHg (right arm)
- Standing BP: 120/80 mmHg at 1 min

Haematological Profile

- Haemoglobin: 14 g/dL
- Haematocrit: 45%
- Fasting plasma glucose: 98 mg/dL
- Lipid profile: TOT-C, 134 mg/dL; LDL-C, 72.6 mg/dL; HDL-C, 45 mg/dL; TG, 82 mg/dL
- Electrolytes: sodium, 143 mEq/L; potassium, 4.0 mEq/L
- Serum uric acid: 6.4 mg/dL
- Renal function: urea, 34 mg/dL; creatinine, 0.85 mg/dL; creatinine clearance (Cockroft-Gault), 84.1 mL/min; estimated glomerular filtration rate (eGFR) (MDRD), 102 mL/min/1.73 m^2

Current Treatment

- Telmisartan 80 mg
- Rivaroxaban 20 mg
- Torasemide 10 mg

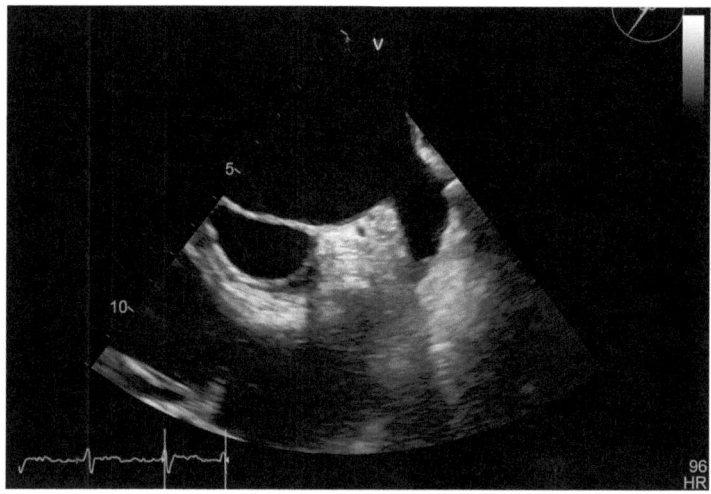

FIGURE 1.4 Transesophageal echocardiography (TEE) showing absence of thrombus in left ventricular appendage

Trans-oesophageal Echocardiogram (TEE)

Absence of thrombus in left ventricular appendage (Fig. 1.4).

Electrical Cardioversion

Three attempts applying energies up to 360 J without having sinus rhythm.

Prescriptions

- Telmisartan 80 mg
- Rivaroxaban 20 mg
- Torasemide 10 mg

1.4   Follow-Up (Visit 3) at 1 Year

At follow-up visit, the patient is asymptomatic for dyspnoea. He continues to practice moderate physical activity two times per week with beneficial effects. He also reports good adherence to prescribed medications without adverse reactions or drug-related side effects.

Physical Examination

- Weight: 76 kg
- Resting pulse: irregular rhythm with normal heart rate, 67 beats/min
- Respiration: normal
- Heart sounds: S1–S2 regular, normal and no murmurs

Blood Pressure Profile

- Home BP (average): 120/70 mmHg
- Sitting BP: 130/80 mmHg (right arm)
- Standing BP: 125/80 mmHg at 1 min

Echocardiogram

Eccentric LV hypertrophy (LV mass indexed 60 g/m^2, relative wall thickness 0.33) with normal chamber dimension (LV end-diastolic diameter 54 mm), normal ejection fraction (LV ejection fraction 59%). Normal dimension of the aortic root and left atrial dilatation (48.08 cm^3/m^2). Right ventricle with normal dimension and function. Pericardium without relevant abnormalities.

Mitral (+) and aortic (+) regurgitations at Doppler ultrasound examination.

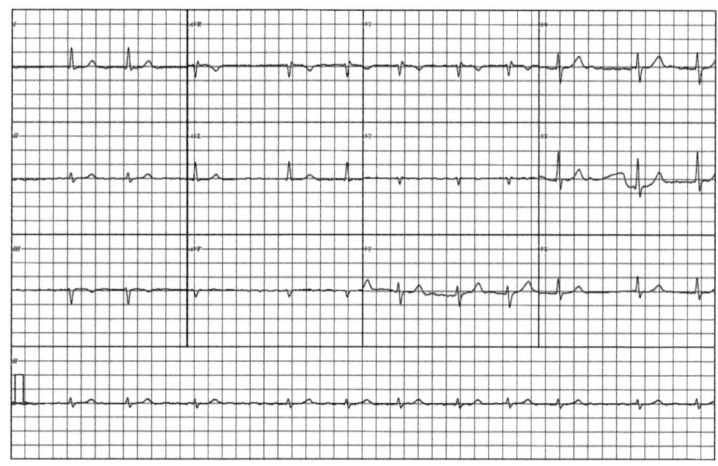

FIGURE 1.5 12-lead electrocardiogram at the last available visit

12-Lead Electrocardiogram

Atrial fibrillation with average heart rate 67 bpm (Fig. 1.5).

Current Treatment

- Telmisartan 80 mg
- Rivaroxaban 20 mg
- Torasemide 10 mg

Prescriptions

- Telmisartan 80 mg
- Rivaroxaban 20 mg
- Torasemide 10 mg

1.5   Discussion

This clinical case describes a patient with controlled blood pressure and presence of cardiac organ damage (left ventricular hypertrophy). According to the 2013 ESH/ESC guidelines on the clinical management of hypertension [1], this patient is classified at high cardiovascular risk. In addition, this patient presents left atrial dilatation. A pathophysiologic consequence of left ventricular hypertrophy and fibrosis is chronic diastolic LV dysfunction, which is associated with left atrial dilatation [2, 3].

In the past decades, a large amount of data has been accumulated on the clinical and prognostic impact of increased left atrial size in human hypertension as a strong, independent predictor of atrial fibrillation [4, 5] and stroke [6, 7]. In a recent study, we identified the risk profile for left atrial (LA) dilatation, characterized by older age, female sex, obesity, higher left ventricular (LV) mass and worse diastolic function.

In this subgroup of patients, the use of diuretics seems to protect against LA dilatation [8]. It is well known that ACE (angiotensin-converting enzyme) inhibitors and angiotensin receptor blockers (ARBs) [9] are able to prevent atrial fibrillation in hypertensive patients. According to these evidences, we prescribed an ARB as antihypertensive therapy.

For the prevention of stroke, we preferred rivaroxaban, both before cardioversion (according to the X-VeRT (*eXplore the efficacy and safety of once-daily oral riVaroxaban for the prevention of caRdiovascular events in patients with non-valvular aTrial fibrillation scheduled for cardioversion*) study) [10] and after failure of cardioversion (according the ROCKET AF (*Rivaroxaban Once Daily Oral Direct Factor Xa Inhibition Compared with Vitamin K Antagonism for Prevention of Stroke and Embolism Trial in Atrial Fibrillation*) trial) [11].

Take-Home Messages
A pathophysiologic consequence of left ventricular hypertrophy and fibrosis is chronic diastolic left ventricular dysfunction, which is associated with left atrial dilatation.

Left atrial size in human hypertension is a potent, independent predictor of atrial fibrillation and stroke.

ACE inhibitors and ARBs are able to prevent atrial fibrillation in hypertensive patients.

Novel oral anticoagulant agents (NOACs) are able to prevent thromboembolic stroke in atrial fibrillation.

References

1. Mancia G, Fagard R, Narkiewicz K, Redon J, Zanchetti A, Bohm M, et al. 2013 ESH/ESC guidelines for the management of arterial hypertension: the task force for the Management of Arterial Hypertension of the European Society of Hypertension (ESH) and of the European Society of Cardiology (ESC). Eur Heart J. 2013;34(28):2159–219.
2. Burlew BS, Weber KT. Cardiac fibrosis as a cause of diastolic dysfunction. Herz. 2002;27(2):92–8.
3. Abhayaratna WP, Seward JB, Appleton CP, Douglas PS, Oh JK, Tajik AJ, et al. Left atrial size: physiologic determinants and clinical applications. J Am Coll Cardiol. 2006;47(12):2357–63.
4. Verdecchia P, Reboldi G, Gattobigio R, Bentivoglio M, Borgioni C, Angeli F, et al. Atrial fibrillation in hypertension: predictors and outcome. Hypertension. 2003;41(2):218–23.
5. Losi MA, Izzo R, De Marco M, Canciello G, Rapacciuolo A, Trimarco V, et al. Cardiovascular ultrasound exploration contributes to predict incident atrial fibrillation in arterial hypertension: the Campania salute network. Int J Cardiol. 2015;199:290–5.
6. Nagarajarao HS, Penman AD, Taylor HA, Mosley TH, Butler K, Skelton TN, et al. The predictive value of left atrial size for incident ischemic stroke and all-cause mortality in African Americans: the atherosclerosis risk in communities (ARIC) study. Stroke. 2008;39(10):2701–6.

7. Gardin JM, McClelland R, Kitzman D, Lima JA, Bommer W, Klopfenstein HS, et al. M-mode echocardiographic predictors of six- to seven-year incidence of coronary heart disease, stroke, congestive heart failure, and mortality in an elderly cohort (the cardiovascular health study). Am J Cardiol. 2001;87(9):1051–7.
8. Losi MA, Izzo R, Canciello G, Giamundo A, Manzi MV, Strisciuglio T, et al. Atrial dilatation development in hypertensive treated patients: the Campania-salute network. Am J Hypertens. 2016;29(9):1077–84.
9. Schneider MP, Hua TA, Böhm M, Wachtell K, Kjeldsen SE, Schmieder RE. Prevention of atrial fibrillation by renin-angiotensin system inhibition. J Am Coll Cardiol. 2010;55(21): 2299–307.
10. Cappato R, Ezekowitz MD, Klein AL, Camm AJ, Ma CS, Le Heuzey JY, et al. Rivaroxaban vs. vitamin K antagonists for cardioversion in atrial fibrillation. Eur Heart J. 2014;35(47): 3346–55.
11. Patel MR, Mahaffey KW, Garg J, Pan G, Singer DE, Hacke W, et al. Rivaroxaban versus warfarin in nonvalvular atrial fibrillation. N Engl J Med. 2011;365(10):883–91.

Clinical Case 2
Patient with Essential Hypertension and Aortic Root Dilatation

2.1 Clinical Case Presentation

A 64-year-old, Caucasian male, was admitted to our outpatient clinic for recent uncontrolled hypertension. He reported a more than 12-year-long clinical history of essential hypertension, initially treated with a combination therapy based on ACE (angiotensin-converting enzyme) inhibitors (ramipril 5 mg) and diuretics (hydrochlorothiazide 12.5 mg).

About 5 years before, for suboptimal blood pressure (BP) control, drug therapy was titrated to ramipril 10 mg and hydrochlorothiazide 25 mg, with satisfactory BP control at home and no relevant side effects or adverse reactions.

About 3 years before, he had been reporting uncontrolled BP levels measured at home. For this reason, his referring physician prescribed amlodipine 5 mg daily in addition to the previous prescribed pharmacological therapy, with mild improvement in BP control.

The patient brought to our attention a recent (2 years earlier) echocardiogram that showed aortic root dilatation (47 mm).

In his medical history he also had diabetes and stage II chronic kidney disease.

R. Izzo, *Hypertension and Cardiac Organ Damage*,
Practical Case Studies in Hypertension Management,
DOI 10.1007/978-3-319-56080-9_2,
© Springer International Publishing AG 2017

His current medications included:

- Metformin 1000 mg daily.
- Acetylsalicylic acid (ASA) 100 mg daily.
- Ramipril 10 mg daily.
- Hydrochlorothiazide 25 mg.
- Amlodipine 5 mg.

Family History

Maternal history of hypertension and paternal history of coronary artery disease. He also has one sibling with hypertension.

Clinical History

He was a previous smoker (more than 20 cigarettes daily) for more than 20 years until the age of 60 years. He has two additional modifiable cardiovascular risk factors: sedentary life habits and obesity. There are no further cardiovascular risk factors or non-cardiovascular diseases.

Physical Examination

- Weight: 83 kg.
- Height: 165 cm.
- Body mass index (BMI): 30.4 kg/m^2.
- Waist circumference: 100 cm.
- Respiration: clear breath sound.
- Heart sounds: early diastolic murmur (II/VI Levine), best heard over the right second intercostal space, radiated towards the apex.

There was no jugular venous distension or hepatojugular reflux.

- Abdomen: his abdomen was soft and non-tender.
- Resting pulse: regular rhythm with heart rate of 95 beats/min.
- Carotid arteries: no murmurs.
- Femoral and foot arteries: symmetrical, absence of oedema.

Haematological Profile

- Haemoglobin: 15 g/dL.
- Haematocrit: 45%.
- Fasting plasma glucose: 147 mg/dL.
- Lipid profile: total cholesterol (TOT-C), 253 mg/dL; low-density lipoprotein cholesterol (LDL-C), 182 mg/dL; high-density lipoprotein cholesterol (HDL-C), 39 mg/dL; triglycerides (TG), 158 mg/dL.
- Electrolytes: sodium 137.9 mEq/L; potassium 4.0 mEq/L.
- Serum uric acid: 6.4 mg/dL.
- Renal function: urea 50 mg/dL, creatinine 1.18 mg/dL; estimated glomerular filtration rate (eGFR) (MDRD): 66.06 mL/min/1.73 m^2.
- Urine analysis (dipstick): normal.
- Normal liver function tests.
- Normal thyroid function tests.

Blood Pressure Profile

- Home BP (average): 160–165/95 mmHg.
- Sitting BP: 160/90 mmHg (right arm); 155/88 mmHg (left arm).
- Standing BP: 155/95 mmHg at 1 min.

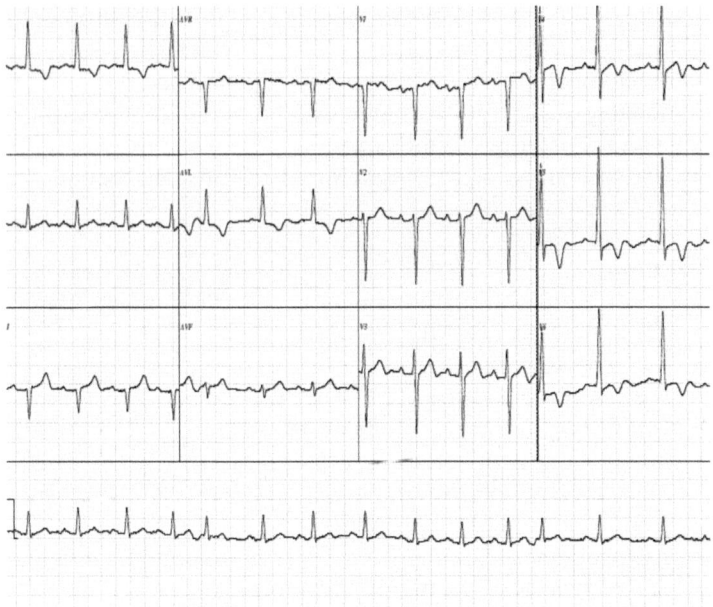

FIGURE 2.1 12-lead ECG at the first available visit

12 Lead ECG

Sinus rhythm with heart rate 90 bpm, normal atrioventricular and intraventricular conduction, ST-segment abnormalities with signs of LVH (Fig. 2.1).

Echocardiogram

Dilatation of ascending aorta with widest diameter at the level of right pulmonary artery, measuring 41 mm. Dilated aortic root, measuring 50 mm. Descending thoracic aorta and pulmonary artery have normal diameters. Left ventricular hypertrophy (LV mass index: 64.5 g/m$^{2.7}$) with eccentric pattern (relative wall thickness [RWT]: 0.36) with left ventricular thickness measured and the left ventricle is not enlarged end diastole (55 mm). There is normal wall motion of 57% and normal diastolic function. Middle aortic regurgitation (Fig. 2.2).

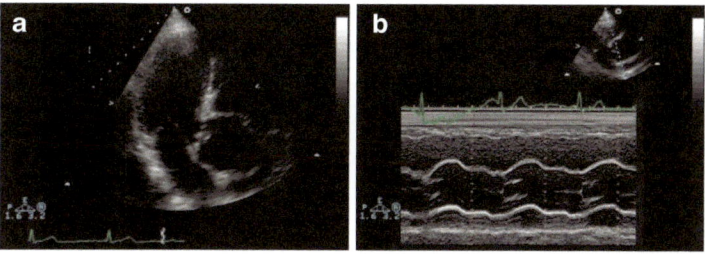

FIGURE 2.2 Echocardiogram at the first visit (Panel a: 5 chamber; panel b: M-mode long axis)

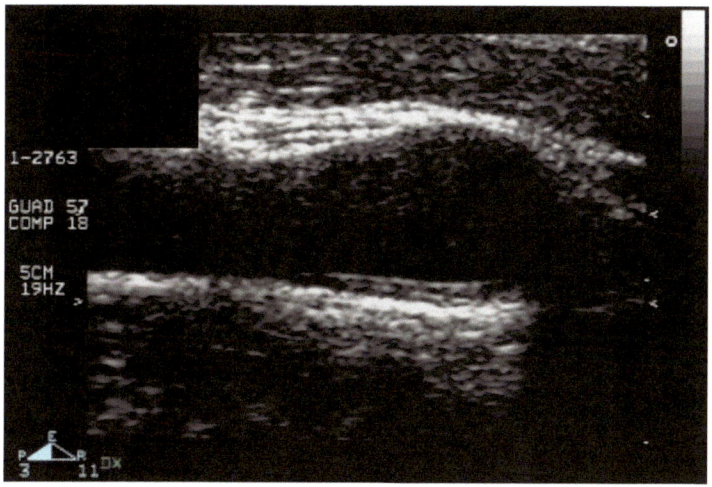

FIGURE 2.3 Carotid ultrasound at the first visit

Vascular Ultrasound

Carotid: intima-media thickness at both carotid levels with evidence of atherosclerotic plaques. At right: atherosclerotic plaque of 2.3 mm extending towards the internal carotid artery (Fig. 2.3).

Diagnosis

Aortic root dilatation in patient with essential hypertension, non-insulin-dependent diabetes and stage II chronic kidney disease, left ventricular hypertrophy, carotid plaque.

Additional modifiable cardiovascular risk factors (sedentary habits and visceral obesity).

Q1: Which is the global cardiovascular risk profile in this patient?
Possible answers are:

1. Low
2. Medium
3. High
4. Very high

Global Cardiovascular Risk Stratification

According to the 2013 European Society of Hypertension (ESH)/European Society of Cardiology (ESC) global cardiovascular risk stratification [1], this patient has very high cardiovascular risk (hypertension + type II diabetes mellitus + stage II chronic kidney disease + left ventricular hypertrophy + carotid plaque).

Treatment Evaluation

- Start bisoprolol 2.5 mg daily.
- Start atorvastatin 20 mg.
- Titrate the dose of amlodipine to 10 mg.

Prescriptions

- Periodical BP evaluation at home according to recommendations from guidelines.
- Low-calorie and low-salt intake.

2.2   Follow-Up (Visit 1) at 6 Weeks

At follow-up visit, the patient is apparently healthy and reports good adherence to prescribed medications, although he experienced drug-related side effects.

Physical Examination

- Weight: 83 kg.
- Waist circumference: 100 cm.
- Resting pulse: regular rhythm with heart rate of 70 beats/min.
- Respiration: normal.
- Heart sounds: early diastolic murmur (II/VI Levine), best heard over the right second intercostal space, radiated towards the apex. There was no jugular venous distension or hepatojugular reflux.
- Femoral and foot arteries: severe oedema of both lower extremities.

Lipid Profile

- TOT-C: 212 mg/dL; LDL-C:162 mg/dL; HDL-C: 37 mg/dL; TG: 165 mg/dL.

Blood Pressure Profile

- Home BP (average): 140/90 mmHg.
- Sitting BP: 145/92 mmHg (left arm).
- Standing BP: 143/95 mmHg at 1 min.

12 Lead ECG

Sinus rhythm with heart rate 70 bpm, normal atrioventricular and intraventricular conduction, ST-segment abnormalities with signs of LVH (Fig. 2.4).

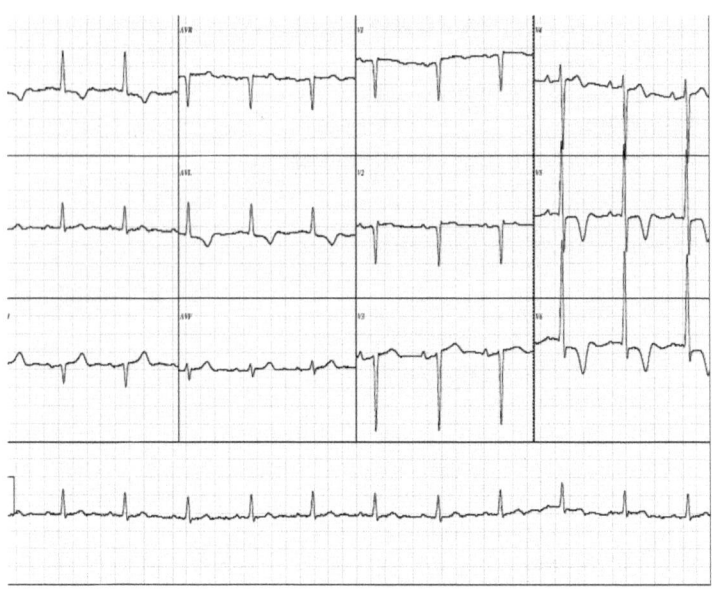

FIGURE 2.4 12-lead ECG at 6 weeks (follow-up visit 1)

Diagnosis

Aortic root dilatation in patient with essential hypertension, non-insulin-dependent diabetes and stage II chronic kidney disease, left ventricular hypertrophy, carotid plaque.

Additional modifiable cardiovascular risk factors (sedentary habits and visceral obesity).

Treatment Evaluation

- Switch from ramipril 10 mg to telmisartan 80 mg.
- Continue hydrochlorothiazide 12.5 mg.

Prescriptions

- A 24-h ambulatory BP monitoring.
- Periodical BP evaluation at home according to recommendations from guidelines.
- Low-calorie and low-salt intake.

2.3   Follow-Up (Visit 2) at 3 Months

At follow-up visit, the patient is in good clinical condition and asymptomatic.

He also reports good adherence to prescribed medications without adverse reactions or drug-related side effects. No relevant changes of the renal function have been documented.

Physical Examination

- Weight: 83 kg.
- Resting pulse: regular rhythm with heart rate of 66 beats/min.
- Respiration: basal crepitations.
- Heart sounds: early diastolic murmur (II/VI Levine), best heard over the right second intercostal space, radiated towards the apex.

Blood Pressure Profile

- Home BP (average): 130/80 mmHg (early morning).
- Sitting BP: 145/85 mmHg (left arm).
- Standing BP: 135/90 mmHg at 1 min.
- 24-h BP: 123/78 mmHg; HR: 62 bpm.
- Daytime BP: 129/82 mmHg; HR: 66 bpm.
- Night-time BP: 110/69 mmHg; HR: 54 bpm.
- 24-h ambulatory BP profile is illustrated in Fig. 2.5.

Lead Electrocardiogram

Sinus rhythm with heart rate 66 bpm, normal atrioventricular and intraventricular conduction, ST-segment abnormalities with signs of LVH.

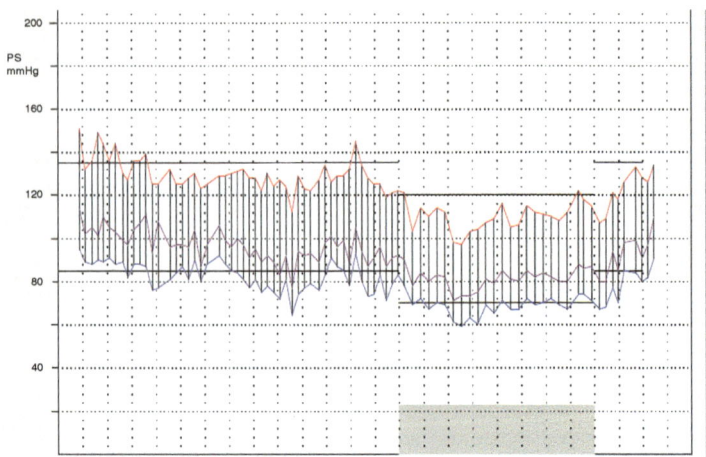

FIGURE 2.5 24-h ambulatory blood pressure profile at 3 months (follow-up visit 2)

Echocardiogram

Dilatation of ascending aorta with widest diameter at level of right pulmonary artery, measuring 44 mm. Dilatation of aortic root, measuring 53 mm. Descending thoracic aorta and pulmonary artery have normal diameters. Left ventricular hypertrophy with eccentric pattern. Left ventricular thickness was measured, and the LV end-diastolic diameter is not enlarged. There is normal wall motion of 59% and normal diastolic function. Middle aortic regurgitation.

CT with Contrast Medium

Aortic root dilatation (50 mm) and ascending aorta dilatation (42 mm).

Diagnosis

Stable aortic root dilatation in patient with essential hypertension, non-insulin-dependent diabetes and stage II chronic kidney disease, left ventricular hypertrophy, carotid plaque.

Additional modifiable cardiovascular risk factors (sedentary habits and visceral obesity).

Treatment Evaluation

- No changes to prescribed therapy.

Prescriptions

- Periodical BP evaluation at home according to recommendations from current guidelines.
- Periodical control of routine chemistry.
- Low-calorie and low-salt intake.

2.4   Follow-Up (Visit 3) at 6 Months

At follow-up visit, the patient is in good clinical condition. He is asymptomatic and has a good control of home BP values.

Physical Examination

- Weight: 86 kg.
- Resting pulse: regular rhythm with heart rate of 61 beats/min.
- Respiration: normal.
- Early diastolic murmur (III/VI Levine) is heard, particularly over the right second intercostal space, radiated towards the apex.

Blood Pressure Profile

- Home BP (average): 125/70 mmHg (early morning).
- Sitting BP: 130/80 mmHg (left arm).
- Standing BP: 127/83 mmHg at 1 min.

Lipid Profile

• TOT-C, 243 mg/dL; LDL-C, 170 mg/dL; HDL-C, 35 mg/dL; TG, 187 mg/dL.

Lead Electrocardiogram

Sinus rhythm with heart rate 60 bpm, normal atrioventricular and intraventricular conduction, ST-segment abnormalities with signs of LVH.

Echocardiogram

Dilatation of ascending aorta (42 mm) and aortic root (49 mm). Descending thoracic aorta and pulmonary artery have normal diameters. Eccentric left ventricular hypertrophy without end-diastolic dilatation. There is normal wall motion of 58% and normal diastolic function. Middle aortic regurgitation.

Diagnosis

Chronic aortic root dilatation in patient with essential hypertension, non-insulin-dependent diabetes and stage II chronic kidney disease, left ventricular hypertrophy, carotid plaque.

Additional modifiable cardiovascular risk factors (sedentary habits and visceral obesity).

Q2: Which is the best therapeutic option in this patient?
Possible answers are:

1. No changes
2. Add another antihypertensive
3. Increase atorvastatin
4. Change telmisartan

Treatment Evaluation

- Lifestyle changes.
- Titrate the dose of atorvastatin to 40 mg.
- No changes to other drugs.

Prescriptions

- Periodical BP evaluation at home according to recommendations from current guidelines
- Periodical control of routine chemistry
- Low-calorie and low-salt intake

2.5   Follow-Up (Visit 4) at 1 Year

At follow-up visit, the patient is in good clinical condition. He experienced dyspnoea for intense efforts, NYHA (New York Health Association) classification II.

Physical Examination

- Weight: 80 kg.
- Resting pulse: regular rhythm with 60 beats/min.
- Absence of peripheral oedema.
- Respiration: normal.
- Heart sounds: an early diastolic murmur (III/VI Levine).

Haematological Profile

- Haemoglobin: 15.1 g/dL.
- Haematocrit: 47%.
- Fasting plasma glucose: 124 mg/dL.
- HbA1C: 42 mmol/mol (6%).
- Lipid profile: TOT-C, 193 mg/dL; LDL-C, 125 mg/dL; HDL-C, 40 mg/dL; TG, 139 mg/dL.

- Electrolytes: sodium, 140 mEq/L; potassium, 3.9 mEq/L.
- Serum uric acid: 6.3 mg/dL.
- Renal function: urea 48 mg/dL, creatinine, 1.1 mg/dL; estimated glomerular filtration rate (eGFR) (MDRD): 67 mL/min/1.73 m^2.
- Urine analysis (dipstick): normal.
- Normal liver function tests.
- Normal thyroid function tests.

Blood Pressure Profile

- Home BP (average): 130/70 mmHg.
- Sitting BP: 130/75 mmHg (left arm).
- Standing BP: 125/75 mmHg at 1 min.

Lead Electrocardiogram

Sinus rhythm with heart rate 60 bpm, normal atrioventricular and intraventricular conduction, ST-segment abnormalities with signs of LVH.

Echocardiogram

The echocardiography showed ascending aorta (41 mm) and aortic root (50 mm) dilatation. Eccentric left ventricular hypertrophy (LV mass indexed 57.1 g/m$^{2.7}$, relative wall thickness 0.38) with normal chamber dimension (LV end-diastolic diameter 52 mm), impaired left ventricular relaxation (E/A ratio < 1) at both conventional and tissue Doppler evaluations and normal ejection fraction (60%). Normal dimension of left atrium. Right ventricle with normal dimension and function. Pericardium without relevant abnormalities.

Mitral (++), tricuspid (+) and aortic (++) regurgitations at Doppler ultrasound examination.

Diagnosis

Chronic aortic root dilatation in patient with essential hypertension, non-insulin-dependent diabetes and stage II chronic kidney disease, left ventricular hypertrophy, carotid plaque.

Current Treatment

- Telmisartan 80 mg.
- Bisoprolol 2.5 mg.
- Metformin 1000 mg daily.
- Hydrochlorotiazide 12.5 mg.
- Amlodipine 10 mg.
- Atorvastatina 40 mg.

Treatment Evaluation

- No changes to the current therapy.

Prescriptions

- Periodical BP evaluation at home according to recommendations from current guidelines.
- Periodical control of routine chemistry.
- Low-calorie and low-salt intake.
- Strict control of aortic root dimension through periodical echocardiographic assessment (every 6 months).

2.6   Discussion

This clinical case describes a patient with essential hypertension, aortic root dilatation, non-insulin-dependent diabetes, left ventricular hypertrophy and carotid atherosclerotic plaque. The 2013 ESH/ESC guidelines on the clinical management of hypertension [1] identify this patient as at high cardiovascular risk for the presence of diabetes, left ventricular hypertrophy and carotid plaque, but do not take into account the aortic root dilatation as a risk factor for cardiovascular events.

Aortic root dilatation has been associated with aortic regurgitation, hypertension, arteriosclerosis and hypertension-related end-organ damage, including increased peripheral resistance, carotid intima-media thickness, evidence of plaque [2] and aortic root dimension indexed to height. Also it has been demonstrated to have a predictive value for the incidence of both nonfatal and fatal cardiovascular events [3]. Furthermore, the ratio between the aortic root area and its height provides independent and improved risk stratification for prediction of death [4].

According to the current guidelines, patients with chronic conditions, such as hypertension, should maintain their BP below 140/90 mmHg, by means of lifestyle changes and—if necessary—using antihypertensive drugs [1]. There is no evidence for the efficacy of specific antihypertensive drug classes in preventing the progression of aortic root dilatation, except for patients with Marfan syndrome. Several reports have showed that the prophylactic use of beta blockers, ACE inhibitors and angiotensin receptor blockers (ARBs) seems to be able to reduce either the progression of the aortic dilatation or the occurrence of complications [5–8].

In our patient, we obtained an optimal control of BP and other risk factors (i.e. diabetes and lipid profile), and we suggested to strictly control aortic root dimensions regularly (every 6 months) through echocardiography.

Take-Home Messages
Aortic root dilatation has been associated with other cardiovascular risk factors.

Aortic root dimension indexed to height is predictive of both incident nonfatal and fatal cardiovascular events.

There is no evidence for the efficacy of particular antihypertensive classes of drugs in preventing the progression of aortic root dilatation.

References

1. Mancia G, Fagard R, Narkiewicz K, Redon J, Zanchetti A, Bohm M, et al. 2013 ESH/ESC guidelines for the management of arterial hypertension: the task force for the Management of Arterial Hypertension of the European Society of Hypertension (ESH) and of the European Society of Cardiology (ESC). Eur Heart J. 2013;34(28):2159–219.

2. de Simone G, Roman MJ, De Marco M, Bella JN, Izzo R, Lee ET, et al. Hemodynamic correlates of abnormal aortic root dimension in an adult population: the strong heart study. J Am Heart Assoc. 2015;4(10):e002309.

3. Cuspidi C, Facchetti R, Bombelli M, Re A, Cairoa M, Sala C, et al. Aortic root diameter and risk of cardiovascular events in a general population: data from the PAMELA study. J Hypertens. 2014;32(9):1879–87.

4. Masri A, Kalahasti V, Svensson LG, Roselli EE, Johnston D, Hammer D, et al. Aortic cross-sectional area/height ratio and outcomes in patients with a trileaflet aortic valve and a dilated aorta. Circulation. 2016;134(22):1724–37.

5. Brady AR, Thompson SG, Fowkes FG, Greenhalgh RM, Powell JT, Participants UKSAT. Abdominal aortic aneurysm expansion: risk factors and time intervals for surveillance. Circulation. 2004;110(1):16–21.

6. Groenink M, den Hartog AW, Franken R, Radonic T, de Waard V, Timmermans J, et al. Losartan reduces aortic dilatation rate in adults with Marfan syndrome: a randomized controlled trial. Eur Heart J. 2013;34(45):3491–500.

7. Chiu HH, Wu MH, Wang JK, Lu CW, Chiu SN, Chen CA, et al. Losartan added to beta-blockade therapy for aortic root dilation in Marfan syndrome: a randomized, open-label pilot study. Mayo Clin Proc. 2013;88(3):271–6.

8. Shores J, Berger KR, Murphy EA, Pyeritz RE. Progression of aortic dilatation and the benefit of long-term beta-adrenergic blockade in Marfan's syndrome. N Engl J Med. 1994;330(19): 1335–41.

Clinical Case 3
Patient with Essential Hypertension and Diastolic Heart Failure

3.1 Clinical Case Presentation

An 82-year-old female was admitted with shortness of breath and exertional dyspnoea. She reported partial relief using more than one pillow under the head in bed during sleep. She also referred history of essential hypertension, hypercholesterolaemia and atrial fibrillation.

Hypertension and hypercholesterolaemia had been diagnosed 13 years before and, at that moment, were, respectively, treated with amlodipine 10 mg and atorvastatin 20 mg/day. Atrial fibrillation had been diagnosed 2 years before and was treated with both bisoprolol 2.5 mg and rivaroxaban 20 mg daily.

She referred several admissions to the emergency department having occurred during the two previous months for shortness of breath at rest. For these reasons, her referring physician additionally prescribed her furosemide 25 mg three times a week, which slightly improved her functional status.

Family History

She has paternal history of stroke and maternal history of hypercholesterolaemia. She also has one sibling with hypertension and myocardial infarction.

R. Izzo, *Hypertension and Cardiac Organ Damage*,
Practical Case Studies in Hypertension Management,
DOI 10.1007/978-3-319-56080-9_3,
© Springer International Publishing AG 2017

Clinical History

She never smoked. She has two additional modifiable cardio-vascular risk factors: sedentary life habits and obesity.

Physical Examination

- Weight: 70 kg.
- Height: 152 cm.
- Body mass index (BMI): 30.3 kg/m^2.
- Waist circumference: 107 cm.
- Respiration: late inspiratory crackles are heard bilaterally in the lower lung field.
- Heart exam: S3 is heard at the apex. A holosystolic murmur (III/VI Levine) is heard best at the apex.
- Physical examination reveals severe oedema of both lower extremities (Fig. 1.1).
- Resting pulse: regular rhythm with normal heart rate (76 beats/min).
- Carotid arteries: no murmurs.
- Femoral and foot arteries: normal peripheral pulses.

Haematological Profile

- Haemoglobin: 11.9 g/dL
- Haematocrit: 38%
- Fasting plasma glucose: 87 mg/dL
- NT pro BNP: 978 pg/mL
- Lipid profile: total cholesterol (TOT-C), 245 mg/dL; low-density lipoprotein cholesterol (LDL-C), 155 mg/dL; high-density lipoprotein cholesterol (HDL-C), 55 mg/dL; triglycerides (TG), 160 mg/dL
- Electrolytes: sodium, 140 mEq/L; potassium, 4 mEq/L
- Serum uric acid: 6.5 mg/dL

- Renal function: urea, 40 mg/dL; creatinine, 0.9 mg/dL; estimated glomerular filtration rate (eGFR) (MDRD), 59.74 mL/min/1.73 m^2
- Urine analysis (dipstick): normal
- Normal liver function tests
- Normal thyroid function tests

Blood Pressure Profile

- Home BP (average): 110/60 mmHg
- Sitting BP: 115/65 mmHg (right arm); 110/60 mmHg (left arm)
- Standing BP: 120/60 mmHg at 1 min

12 Lead ECG

Atrial fibrillation with normal heart rate (70 bpm) (Fig. 3.1).

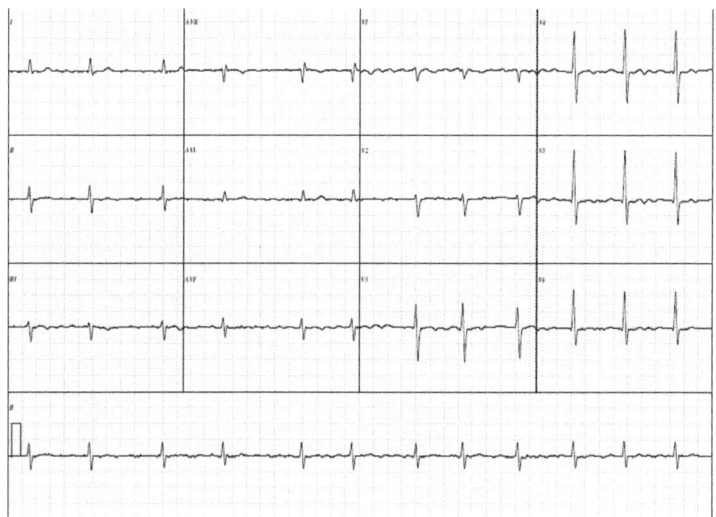

FIGURE 3.1 12 lead ECG at the first available visit

Chest X-Ray

Positive for interstitial oedema.

Echo

Echocardiography showed a concentric hypertrophy (LVMid, 62.7 g/m$^{2.7}$; RWT, 0.5), atrial enlargement (LAVi 50.35 cm^3/m^2) with normal ejection fraction of 55%. Mild mitral and aortic regurgitations. Severe increase in pulmonary systolic blood pressure and increased filling pressures (E/E' ratio 24) (Figs. 3.2 and 3.3).

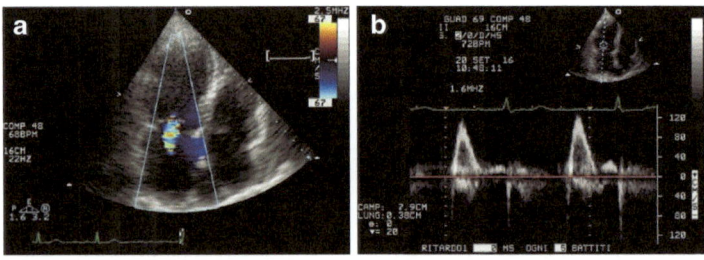

FIGURE 3.2 Echocardiography at the first available visit (Panel a: 4 chamber; panel b: doppler study of mitral valve)

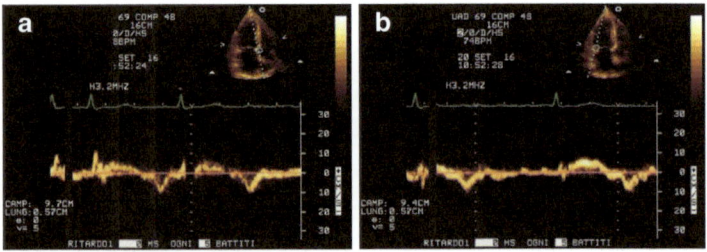

FIGURE 3.3 Echocardiography at the first available visit (Panel a: TDI [tissue doppler imaging] at septum level; panel b: TDI at lateral wall)

Q1: Which is the correct diagnosis?

1. Essential hypertension without heart failure
2. Essential hypertension whit systolic heart failure
3. Essential hypertension with systolic heart failure and atrial fibrillation
4. Essential hypertension with diastolic heart failure and atrial fibrillation

Diagnosis

Diastolic heart failure NYHA (New York Health Association) classification II in patient with essential hypertension, hypercholesterolaemia and atrial fibrillation. Additional modifiable cardiovascular risk factors (sedentary habits and visceral obesity).

Treatment Evaluation

- Start ACE (angiotensin-converting enzyme) inhibitors: ramipril 10 mg daily.
- Stop amlodipine 10 mg.
- Start furosemide 25 mg daily.

Prescriptions

- Periodical BP evaluation at home according to recommendations from guidelines
- Regular physical activity and low-salt intake
- Periodical evaluation for renal function

3.2   Follow-Up (Visit 1) at 6 Weeks

At follow-up visit the patient presents a deterioration of her functional status, having the dyspnoea worsened and being it accompanied by a dry, 3-week-lasting, persistent cough. The cough interferes with her ability to sleep at night and with routine activities during the day. No recent chest infection can explain the cough. She also reports poor adherence to prescribed medications. No significant changes of renal function have been recorded.

Physical Examination

- Weight: 69 kg.
- Resting pulse: irregular rhythm with normal heart rate, 68 beats/min.
- Respiration: no signs of fluid overload.
- Heart sounds: a grade 2/6 holosystolic murmur is heard best at the apex.

Lipid Profile

- TOT-C, 208 mg/dL; LDL-C, 123 mg/dL; HDL-C, 54 mg/dL; TG, 155 mg/dL
- Electrolytes: sodium 143 mEq/L; potassium 4.1 mEq/L
- Serum uric acid: 6.5 mg/dL
- Renal function: urea, 43 mg/dL; creatinine, 1 mg/dL; estimated glomerular filtration rate (eGFR) (MDRD), 52.59 mL/min/1.73 m^2

Blood Pressure Profile

- Home BP (average): 110/65 mmHg
- Sitting BP: 122/70 mmHg (left arm)
- Standing BP: 110/75 mmHg at 1 min

Chest X-Ray

Normal examination.

Diagnosis

Diastolic heart failure (NYHA Class II) in patient with essential hypertension, hypercholesterolaemia and atrial fibrillation.

Additional modifiable cardiovascular risk factors (sedentary habits and visceral obesity).

Treatment Evaluation

- Stop ramipril 10 mg.
- Start losartan 50 mg daily.

Prescriptions

- Periodical BP evaluation at home according to recommendations from guidelines
- Regular physical activity and low-salt intake
- Periodical evaluation for renal function

3.3   Follow-Up (Visit 2) at 3 Months

At follow-up visit, the patient reports increased breathlessness. She also reports good adherence to prescribed medications without adverse reactions or drug-related side effects.

Physical Examination

- Weight: 68 kg.
- Resting pulse: irregular rhythm; heart rate, 71 beats/min.

- Respiration: inspiratory crackles are heard bilaterally in the lower lung field.
- Heart sounds: a holosystolic murmur 2/6 is heard best at the apex.
- BP: 125/70 mmHg.

Renal Function

- Electrolytes: sodium 140 mEq/L; potassium 4 mEq/L
- Renal function: urea, 45 mg/dL; creatinine, 1 mg/dL; estimated glomerular filtration rate (eGFR) (MDRD), 52.59 mL/min/1.73 m^2

Treatment Evaluation

- Start eplerenone 25 mg three times a week.

Prescriptions

- Periodical BP evaluation at home according to recommendations from current guidelines.
- Periodical evaluation for electrolytes and renal function.

3.4   Follow-Up (Visit 3) at 6 Months

At follow-up visit, the patient is in good clinical condition, having NYHA class II.

Physical Examination

- Weight: 69 kg.
- Resting pulse: irregular rhythm with 70 beats/min.
- Absence of peripheral oedema (bilateral).
- Respiration: basal fine crepitation.
- Heart sounds: a holosystolic murmur (II/VI Levine) is heard best at the apex.

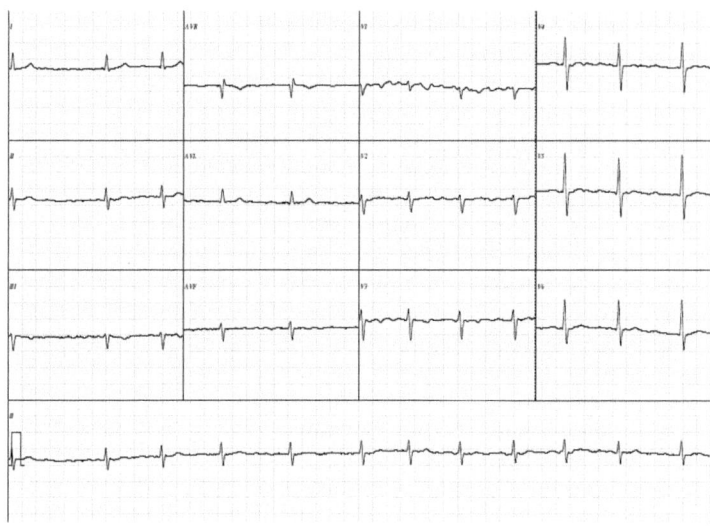

FIGURE 3.4 12-lead ECG at 6 months (follow-up visit 3)

Blood Pressure Profile

- Home BP (average): 120/80 mmHg
- Sitting BP: 127 m/71 mmHg (left arm)
- Standing BP: 124/68 mmHg at 1 min

12 Lead ECG

Atrial fibrillation with normal heart rate (63 bpm), normal intraventricular conduction and ST-segment abnormalities (Fig. 3.4).

Echo

Echocardiography shows a concentric hypertrophy with normal ejection fraction of 55% (LVM indexed: 67.4 g/m$^{2.7}$; RWT: 0.48). Mild mitral and aortic regurgitation. Moderate increase in pulmonary systolic blood pressure and increased filling pressures (E/E' 18).

Current Treatment

- Losartan 50 mg/die
- Bisoprolol 2.5 mg/die

Q2: Which is the best therapeutic option for this patient?

1. Possible answers are:
2. Change losartan with ramipril.
3. Add amlodipine.
4. Stop furosemide.
5. No changes.

- Furosemide 25 mg/die
- Atorvastatin 20 mg/die
- Eplerenone 25 mg three times a week
- Rivaroxaban 20 mg/die

Treatment Evaluation

- No changes in current pharmacological therapy.

Prescriptions

- Periodical BP evaluation at home according to recommendations from current guidelines
- Regular physical activity and low-salt intake
- Periodical evaluation of electrolytes and renal function

3.5   Follow-Up (Visit 4) at 1 Year

At follow-up visit, the patient is in good clinical condition, having NYHA class II.

Physical Examination

- Weight: 70 kg.
- Resting pulse: irregular rhythm with 67 beats/min.
- Absence of peripheral oedema (bilateral).
- Respiration: normal.
- Heart sounds: a grade 2/6 holosystolic murmur is heard best at the apex.

Haematological Profile

- Haemoglobin: 11.5 g/dL
- Hematocrit: 40%
- Fasting plasma glucose: 92 mg/dL
- Lipid profile: TOT-C, 197 mg/dL; LDL-C, 117 mg/dL; HDL-C, 50 mg/dL; TG, 149 mg/dL
- Electrolytes: sodium, 142 mEq/L; potassium, 4.5 mEq/L
- Serum uric acid: 6.8 mg/dL
- Renal function: urea, 50 mg/dL; creatinine, 0.9 mg/dL; estimated glomerular filtration rate (eGFR) (MDRD), 59.32 mL/min/1.73 m^2
- Urine analysis (dipstick): normal
- Normal liver function tests
- Normal thyroid function tests

Blood Pressure Profile

- Home BP (average): 118/65 mmHg
- Sitting BP: 123/67 mmHg (left arm)
- Standing BP: 120/71 mmHg at 1 min

Lead Electrocardiogram

Atrial fibrillation with normal heart rate (63 bpm), normal intraventricular conduction and ST-segment abnormalities.

Treatment Evaluation

• No changes in current pharmacological therapy.

Prescriptions

• Periodical BP evaluation at home according to recommendations from current guidelines
• Regular physical activity and low-salt intake
• Periodical evaluation for electrolytes and renal function

3.6   Discussion

Arterial hypertension is the most common cardiovascular risk factor and the principal precursor of heart failure [1]. Diastolic dysfunction might represent an important pathophysiological intermediate between hypertension and heart failure [2]. Diastolic dysfunction is part of a clinical syndrome characterized by symptoms and signs of heart failure with a preserved ejection fraction (EF). Diastolic heart failure occurs when the ventricular chamber is unable to accept an adequate volume of blood during diastole, at normal diastolic pressures and at volumes sufficient to maintain an appropriate stroke volume [3].

Diastolic dysfunction has significant pathological effects on both atrial structure and function, many of which are proarrhythmic (i.e. atrial fibrillation) [4], and the onset of atrial fibrillation worsens the symptoms of heart failure.

Diuretic-based antihypertensive therapy, ACE inhibitors, ARBs and beta blockers are also effective in reducing symptoms and progression of diastolic dysfunction in hypertensive patients with diastolic dysfunction [5]. Diuretics should be prescribed to all patients who have evidence of fluid retention. Diuretics should generally be combined with an ACE inhibitor, ARBs, beta blocker and aldosterone antagonist.

Finally, beta blockers have been demonstrated to reduce mortality in patients with diastolic dysfunction and are therefore currently recommended to all patients with heart failure, especially for heart rate control in case of atrial fibrillation [6].

Take-Home Messages
Arterial hypertension is the most common risk factor for heart failure.

Diastolic dysfunction is part of a clinical syndrome characterized by symptoms and signs of heart failure with a preserved ejection fraction.

Echocardiography represents the gold standard for the diagnosis of diastolic dysfunction.

Diuretic-based antihypertensive therapy, ACE inhibitors, ARBs and beta blockers are also effective in reducing symptoms and progression of diastolic dysfunction.

References

1. Levy D, Larson MG, Vasan RS, Kannel WB, Ho KK. The progression from hypertension to congestive heart failure. JAMA. 1996;275(20):1557–62.
2. Solomon SD, Janardhanan R, Verma A, Bourgoun M, Daley WL, Purkayastha D, et al. Effect of angiotensin receptor blockade and antihypertensive drugs on diastolic function in patients with hypertension and diastolic dysfunction: a randomised trial. Lancet. 2007;369(9579):2079–87.

3. Zile MR, Brutsaert DL. New concepts in diastolic dysfunction and diastolic heart failure: part I: diagnosis, prognosis, and measurements of diastolic function. Circulation. 2002;105(11):1387–93.
4. Rosenberg MA, Manning WJ. Diastolic dysfunction and risk of atrial fibrillation: a mechanistic appraisal. Circulation. 2012; 126(19):2353–62.
5. Yancy CW, Jessup M, Bozkurt B, Butler J, Casey DE, Drazner MH, et al. 2013 ACCF/AHA guideline for the Management of Heart Failure: executive summary. A report of the American College of Cardiology Foundation/American Heart Association task force on practice guidelines. Circulation. 2013;128(16): 1810–52.
6. David D, Segni ED, Klein HO, Kaplinsky E. Inefficacy of digitalis in the control of heart rate in patients with chronic atrial fibrillation: beneficial effect of an added beta adrenergic blocking agent. Am J Cardiol. 1979;44(7):1378–82.

Clinical Case 4
Patient with Essential Hypertension and Systolic Heart Failure

4.1 Clinical Case Presentation

A 74-year-old Caucasian male was admitted to the outpatient clinic for recent shortness of breath.

Over the previous 5 months, he reported increased shortness of breath and fatigue after a steady 10 min walk at the park. Since then, he reduced his level of physical activity. He is used to sleep with two, sometimes three, pillows. He did not report having experienced chest pain, leg pain or fainting spells.

He was diagnosed with heart failure 1 year before (LVEF 38%) and, after a myocardial infarction, treated with a coronary-artery bypass. He also referred history of essential hypertension and diabetes treated with oral medications.

His therapy included:

- Ramipril 2.5 mg
- Atenolol 50 mg
- Furosemide 20 mg (three times a week)
- Acetylsalicylic acid (ASA) 100 mg
- Atorvastatin 20 mg
- Metformin 500 mg (three times a day)

R. Izzo, *Hypertension and Cardiac Organ Damage,*
Practical Case Studies in Hypertension Management,
DOI 10.1007/978-3-319-56080-9_4,
© Springer International Publishing AG 2017

Family History

He has paternal history of hypertension and myocardial infarction and maternal history of diabetes and hypercholesterolaemia. He also has one sibling with hypertension and stroke.

Clinical History

Former smoker (about 10–20 cigarettes daily) for more than 40 years, non-smoker for 1 year at presentation to the clinic. He also has two additional modifiable cardiovascular risk factors: sedentary life habits and overweight (visceral obesity). There are no further cardiovascular risk factors, associated clinical conditions or non-cardiovascular diseases.

Physical Examination

- Weight: 89 kg.
- Height: 171 cm.
- Body mass index (BMI): 30.44 kg/m^2.
- Waist circumference: 121 cm.
- Respiration: inspiratory crackles are heard bilaterally in the lower lung field.
- Heart exam: S1–S2 are diminished. S3 is heard at the apex. A grade 3/6 holosystolic murmur is heard best at the apex; it radiated to the left axilla.
- There is oedema of both lower extremities.
- Examination of the abdomen: The anterior wall is round and soft. The liver edge is palpable. The spleen is not palpable.
- Resting pulse: regular rhythm with normal heart rate of 67 beats/min.
- Carotid arteries: no murmurs.
- Femoral and foot arteries: diminished peripheral pulses.

Haematological Profile

- Haemoglobin: 14.4 g/dL
- Haematocrit: 45%
- Fasting plasma glucose: 117 mg/dL
- NT pro BNP: 897 pg/mL
- Lipid profile: total cholesterol (TOT-C), 184 mg/dL; low-density lipoprotein cholesterol (LDL-C), 115 mg/dL; high-density lipoprotein cholesterol (HDL-C), 39 mg/dL; triglycerides (TG), 147 mg/dL
- Electrolytes: sodium, 146 mEq/L; potassium, 4.2 mEq/L
- Serum uric acid: 4.1 mg/dL
- Renal function: urea, 24 mg/dL; creatinine, 0.8 mg/dL; estimated glomerular filtration rate (eGFR) (MDRD), 88 mL/min/1.73 m^2
- Urine analysis (dipstick): normal
- Albuminuria: 12.2 mg/24 h
- Normal liver function tests
- Normal thyroid function tests

Blood Pressure Profile

- Home BP (average): 145/90 mmHg
- Sitting BP: 155/95 mmHg (right arm); 150/93 mmHg (left arm)
- Standing BP: 152/98 mmHg at 1 min

Lead Electrocardiogram

Sinus rhythm with normal heart rate (63 bpm) with anterolateral Q waves (signs of previous infarction). Normal atrioventricular and intraventricular conduction.

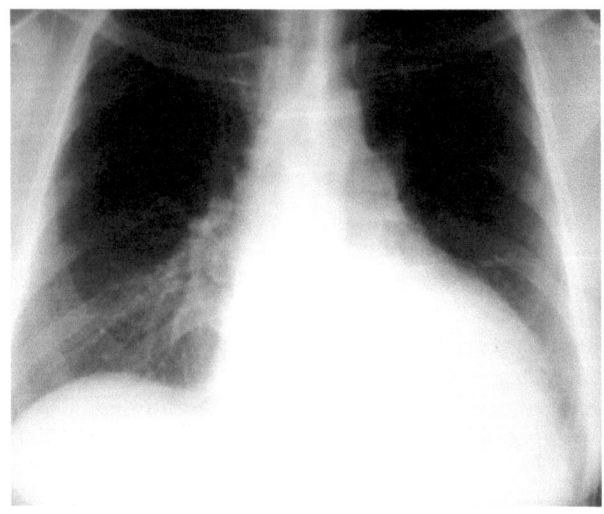

FIGURE 4.1 Chest X-ray at the first visit

Chest X-Ray

There is moderate cardiac enlargement. Pulmonary vascular congestion and mild pulmonary oedema are present: increased haziness and decreased radiolucency of the lung parenchyma bilaterally (Fig. 4.1).

Echocardiography

The echocardiogram showed a dilated heart; in particular, the following diameters have been recorded: left ventricular end-diastolic dimension 61 cm, left ventricular end-systolic dimension 50 cm. In addition, anterior and septal hypokinesis associated with apical dilatation and reduced left ventricular ejection fraction (28%) as a marker of previous anterior infarction were found. Finally, mild mitral regurgitation was detected (Fig. 4.2).

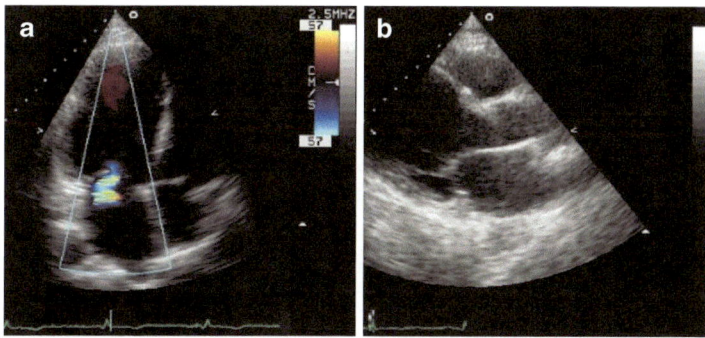

Figure 4.2 Echocardiography at the first visit (Panel a: 4 chamber; panel b: long axis)

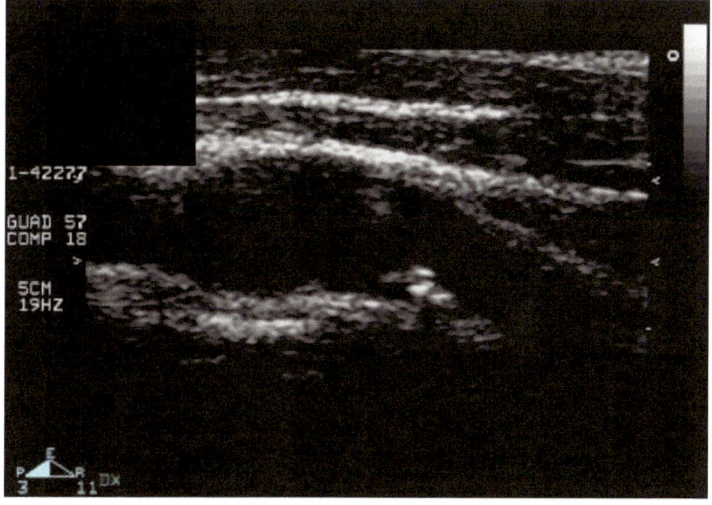

Figure 4.3 Carotid ultrasound at the first visit

Vascular Ultrasound

Carotid: intima-media thickness at both carotid levels (at right, atherosclerotic plaque extending towards the internal carotid artery) with evidence of atherosclerotic plaques (Fig. 4.3).

Diagnosis

Systolic heart failure New York Health Association (NYHA) class III in patient with ischaemic dilated cardiomyopathy, essential hypertension and non-insulin-dependent diabetes.

Additional modifiable cardiovascular risk factors (sedentary habits and visceral obesity).

Treatment Evaluation

- Titrate the dose of ACE inhibitor ramipril from 2.5 to 5 mg.
- Titrate the dose of atorvastatin from 20 to 40 mg.
- Switch from atenolol to bisoprolol 2.5 mg daily.
- Start furosemide 25 mg every day.

Prescriptions

- Periodical BP evaluation at home according to recommendations from guidelines
- Low-calorie and low-salt intake

4.2   Follow-Up (Visit 1) at 6 Weeks

At follow-up visit, the patient is in good clinical condition. No increase in dyspnoea with reduction of ankle oedema. No significant changes of renal function were documented.

He also reports good adherence to prescribed medications without adverse reactions or drug-related side effects.

Physical Examination

- Weight: 87 kg.
- Waist circumference: 119 cm.
- Resting pulse: regular rhythm; heart rate, 65 beats/min.
- Respiration: Basal fine crepitation.
- Heart sounds: a holosystolic murmur (III/VI Levine) is heard best at the apex; it radiated to the left axilla.

Lipid Profile

- TOT-C: 134 mg/dL.
- LDL-C: 70 mg/dL.
- HDL-C: 40 mg/dL.
- TG: 117 mg/dL.

Blood Pressure Profile

- Home BP (average): 130/85 mmHg
- Sitting BP: 148/92 mmHg (left arm)
- Standing BP: 145/95 mmHg at 1 min

Lead Electrocardiogram

Sinus rhythm with normal heart rate (68 bpm) with anterolateral Q waves of previous infarction. Normal atrioventricular and intraventricular conduction.

Diagnosis

Systolic heart failure (NYHA class II) in patient with isch-aemic dilated cardiomyopathy and non-insulin-dependent diabetes.

Additional modifiable cardiovascular risk factors (seden-tary habits and visceral obesity).

Treatment Evaluation

- Titrate the dose of ramipril from 5 to 10 mg.
- Start canrenone 25 mg three times a week.

4.3   Follow-Up (Visit 2) at 3 Months

At follow-up visit, the patient is in good clinical condition, having NYHA class II. No significant changes of the renal function were documented.

Physical Examination

- Weight: 86 kg.
- Resting pulse: regular rhythm; heart rate, 61 beats/min.
- Respiration: Basal fine crepitations.
- A holosystolic murmur (III/VI Levine) is heard best at the apex; it radiated to the left axilla.
- BP: 125/70 mmHg.

Echo and RM

Dilated heart with reduced left ventricular ejection fraction (31%) and mild mitral regurgitation.

Q2: Which is the best therapeutic option in this patient?
Possible answers are:

1. No changes.
2. Stop canrenone.
3. Stop furosemide.
4. Implantable cardioverter defibrillators (ICDs).

Treatment Evaluation

- Implantable ICDs.

Prescriptions

- Periodical BP evaluation at home according to recommendations from current guidelines
- Periodical control visit for ICDs
- Periodical control of routine chemistry

4.4   Follow-Up (Visit 3) at 1 Year

At follow-up visit, the patient is in good clinical condition. He reports dyspnoea in the case of intense efforts (NYHA II).

Physical Examination

- Weight: 86 kg
- Resting pulse: regular rhythm with 60 beats/min
- Absence of peripheral oedema
- Respiration: normal
- Heart sounds: a holosystolic murmur (III/VI Levine) at the apex

Haematological Profile

- Haemoglobin: 15.1 g/dL
- Haematocrit: 47%
- Fasting plasma glucose: 124 mg/dL
- Lipid profile: TOT-C, 137 mg/dL; LDL-C, 70 mg/dL; HDL-C, 44 mg/dL; TG, 115 mg/dL
- Electrolytes: sodium, 143 mEq/L; potassium, 4.4 mEq/L
- Serum uric acid: 6 mg/dL
- Renal function: urea, 24 mg/dL; creatinine, 0.9 mg/dL; estimated glomerular filtration rate (eGFR) (MDRD), 83.26 mL/min/1.73 m^2
- Urine analysis (dipstick): normal
- Normal liver function tests
- Normal thyroid function tests

Blood Pressure Profile

- Home BP (average): 125/80 mmHg
- Sitting BP: 130/80 mmHg (left arm)
- Standing BP: 128/86 mmHg at 1 min

Lead Electrocardiogram

Sinus rhythm with normal heart rate (63 bpm) with anterolateral Q waves, as a marker of previous infarction. Normal atrioventricular and intraventricular conduction.

ICD Control

Absence of major arrhythmic events.

Chest X-Ray

There is moderate cardiac enlargement. Evidence of ICD.

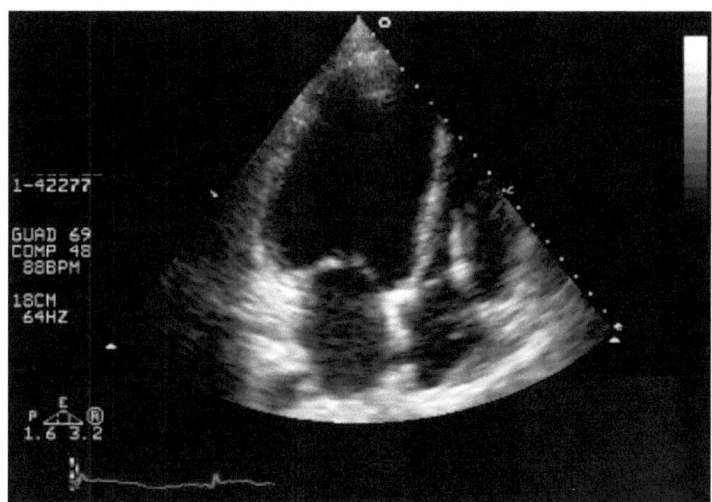

FIGURE 4.4 Echocardiography at 1 year (follow-up visit 3)

Echocardiography

The echocardiography showed a dilated heart with anterior and septal hypokinesis and apical dilatation. Ejection fraction, 30%; mild mitral regurgitation. Evidence of ICD (Fig. 4.4).

Current Treatment

- Ramipril 10 mg
- Bisoprolol 2.5 mg
- Furosemide 25 mg
- Canrenone 25 mg three times a week
- Acetylsalicylic acid 100 mg
- Atorvastatin 40 mg
- Metformin 500 mg three times a day

Treatment Evaluation

- No changes to current pharmacological therapy

Prescriptions

- Periodical BP evaluation at home according to recommendations from current guidelines
- Regular physical activity and low-salt intake
- Periodical control visit for ICDs
- Periodical control of routine chemistry

4.5   Discussion

Hypertension represents the most important modifiable risk factor for heart failure and coronary artery disease (CAD). CAD with previous myocardial infarction (MI) is a major cause of heart failure with reduced ejection fraction [1].

A trial included in a diuretic-based programme demonstrated a number needed to treat of 52 to prevent one heart failure event in 2 years [2]. In another study, elderly patients with previous myocardial infarction had a >80% risk reduction for incident heart failure with tight BP control [3]. Diuretic-based antihypertensive therapy has repeatedly been shown to prevent heart failure in a wide range of patients; ACE inhibitors, ARBs and beta blockers are also effective [1, 4].

ICD therapy is recommended for primary prevention of sudden cardiac death to reduce total mortality in selected patients with non-ischaemic dilated cardiomyopathy or ischaemic heart disease at least 40 days post-myocardial infarction with left ventricular ejection fraction of 35% or less and NYHA class II or III symptoms [5].

Take-Home Messages

Hypertension represents the most important modifiable risk factor for heart failure and coronary artery disease.

Coronary artery disease with previous myocardial infarction is a major cause of heart failure with reduced ejection fraction.

Diuretics, ACE inhibitors, ARBs and beta blockers are effective in preventing heart failure, and diuretic-based antihypertensive therapy has repeatedly been shown to prevent early stages of heart failure and progression towards end-stage congestive heart failure.

ICD therapy is recommended for primary prevention of sudden cardiac death in specific subsets of patients.

References

1. Yancy CW, Jessup M, Bozkurt B, Butler J, Casey Jr DE, et al. 2013 ACCF/AHA guideline for the management of heart failure: a report of the American College of Cardiology Foundation/ American Heart Association task force on practice guidelines. Circulation. 2013;128(16):e240–327.
2. Beckett NS, Peters R, Fletcher AE, Staessen JA, Liu L, Dumitrascu D, et al. Treatment of hypertension in patients 80 years of age or older. N Engl J Med. 2008;358(18):1887–98.
3. Kostis JB, Davis BR, Cutler J, Grimm Jr RH, Berge KG, Cohen JD, et al. Prevention of heart failure by antihypertensive drug treatment in older persons with isolated systolic hypertension. SHEP Cooperative Research Group. JAMA. 1997;278(3):212–6.
4. Gattis WA, O'Connor CM, Gallup DS, Hasselblad V, Gheorghiade M, Investigators I-H, et al. Predischarge initiation of carvedilol in patients hospitalized for decompensated heart failure: results of the Initiation Management Predischarge: Process for Assessment of Carvedilol Therapy in Heart Failure (IMPACT-HF) trial. J Am Coll Cardiol. 2004;43(9):1534–41.
5. Bardy GH, Lee KL, Mark DB, Poole JE, Packer DL, Boineau R, et al. Amiodarone or an implantable cardioverter-defibrillator for congestive heart failure. N Engl J Med. 2005;352(3):225–37.

Clinical Case 5
Patient with Essential Hypertension and Left Ventricular Enlargement

5.1 Clinical Case Presentation

A 51-year-old Caucasian male farmer was admitted to the outpatient clinic reporting a more than 2-year-long clinical history of uncontrolled essential hypertension and mild exertional dyspnoea. The average values of home blood pressure (BP) were 180/100 mmHg.

Family History

Both his parents (84-year-old mother and 85-year-old father) and one brother (61 years old) are hypertensive.

Clinical History

Former smoker (about 20 cigarettes per day from the age of 14 to the age of 45), heavy drinker (about 1 L/day), consuming a diet rich in saturated fats and salt. Works about 12 h/day.

Arterial hypertension has been diagnosed 2 years before. His general practitioner prescribed an antihypertensive

R. Izzo, *Hypertension and Cardiac Organ Damage*, 61
Practical Case Studies in Hypertension Management,
DOI 10.1007/978-3-319-56080-9_5,
© Springer International Publishing AG 2017

therapy based on a fixed combination of atenolol/chlorthalidone 100/25 mg, early interrupted after 1 month for drug-related side effects (erectile dysfunction).

Comorbidities

No other comorbidities or known cardiovascular risk factors, associated clinical conditions or non-cardiovascular diseases were reported.

Physical Examination

- Weight: 94 kg
- Height: 173 cm
- Body mass index (BMI): 31.4 kg/m^2
- Waist circumference: 115 cm
- Respiration: normal
- Heart exam: S1–S2 regular, normal and no murmurs
- Resting pulse: regular rhythm with normal heart rate (72 beats/min)
- Carotid arteries exam: no murmurs
- Femoral and foot arteries: palpable

Haematological Profile

- Haemoglobin: 15.1 g/dL
- Haematocrit: 45.2%
- Fasting plasma glucose: 117 mg/dL
- Lipid profile: total cholesterol (TOT-C): 238 mg/dL; low-density lipoprotein cholesterol (LDL-C): 151.4 mg/dL; high-density lipoprotein cholesterol (HDL-C): 61 mg/dL; triglycerides (TG): 128 mg/dL
- Serum electrolytes: sodium, 143 mEq/L; potassium, 4.8 mEq/L
- Serum uric acid: 4.6 mg/dL
- Renal function: urea, 50 mg/dL; creatinine, 0.98 mg/dL; creatinine clearance (Cockroft-Gault), 122.3 mL/min;

estimated glomerular filtration rate (eGFR) (MDRD), 103 mL/min/1.73 m^2
- Urine analysis (dipstick): normal
- Albuminuria: 10.8 mg/24 h
- Normal liver function tests
- Normal thyroid function tests

Blood Pressure Profile

- Home BP (average): 184/115 mmHg
- Sitting BP: 180/118 mmHg (right arm); 178/116 mmHg (left arm)
- Standing BP: 176/120 mmHg at 1 min

12-Lead ECG

Sinus rhythm with normal heart rate (70 bpm), prolonged atrioventricular conduction (P-R interval 240 ms), criteria for left ventricular hypertrophy (R(I) + S(III) > 2.00 mV), abnormal repolarization in infero-lateral leads (Fig. 5.1).

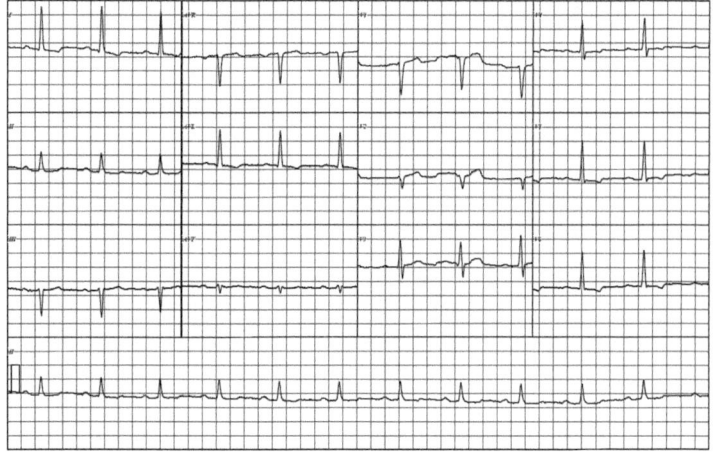

FIGURE 5.1 12-lead ECG at the first available visit

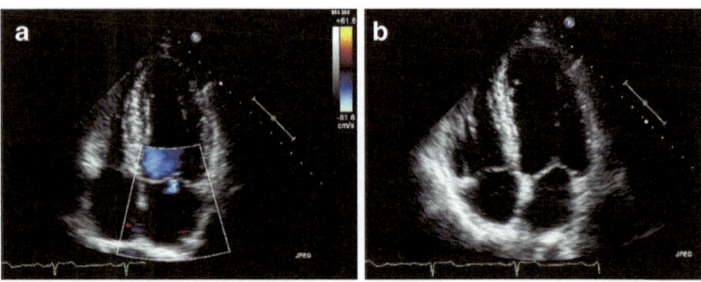

FIGURE 5.2 Echocardiogram at the first visit (Panel a: 4 chamber with color; panel b: 4 chamber without color)

Echocardiogram

Eccentric left ventricular hypertrophy (LV max index 59.3 $g/m^{2.7}$; relative wall thickness 0.33) with high left ventricular chamber dimension (LV end-diastolic diameter 57 mm) and volume (87.19 cm^3/m^2), normal ejection fraction (61%), dilated aortic root (43 mm), normal left atrium, no signs of right ventricle and/or pericardium disease. Aortic (++) regurgitation at Doppler ultrasound examination (Fig. 5.2).

Carotid Ultrasound

Both common carotids presented an increase of intima-media thickness (right, 1.0 mm; left, 0.9 mm) without evidence of significant atherosclerotic plaques.

Current Treatment

The patient does not take any medication.

Diagnosis

Essential (stage III) hypertension with hypertension-related target organ damage (left ventricular hypertrophy), hypercholesterolemia, impaired fasting glucose.

Q1: Which is the global cardiovascular risk profile in this patient?
Possible answers are:

1. Low
2. Medium
3. High
4. Very high

Global Cardiovascular Risk Stratification

According to 2013 European Society of Hypertension (ESH)/ European Society of Cardiology (ESC) global cardiovascular risk stratification [1], this patient has very high cardiovascular risk (grade 3 HTN + 1 asymptomatic organ damage).

Treatment Evaluation

- Start olmesartan 40 mg + amlodipine 5 mg in a single pill.
- Start atorvastatin 20 mg.

Prescriptions

- Periodical BP evaluation at home according to recommendations from current guidelines
- Regular physical activity and low-calorie and low-salt intake

5.2   Follow-Up (Visit 1) After 6 Weeks

At follow-up visit the patient is in good clinical condition. He is regularly practising physical activity and following a low-calorie diet. Mean values of BP at home are normal.

Physical Examination

- Weight: 90 kg
- Body mass index (BMI): 30 kg/m^2
- Resting pulse: regular rhythm with normal heart rate (72 beats/min)
- Other clinical parameters substantially unchanged

Blood Pressure Profile

- Home BP (average): 120/85 mmHg
- Sitting BP: 130/88 mmHg
- Standing BP: 128/88 mmHg

Current Treatment

- Olmesartan 40 mg + amlodipine 5 mg
- Atorvastatin 20 mg

Diagnostic Tests for Organ Damage or Associated Clinical Conditions

No other tests were prescribed.

Diagnosis

Essential (stage III) hypertension with hypertension-related target organ damage (left ventricular hypertrophy), hypercholesterolemia, impaired fasting glucose.

Global Cardiovascular Risk Stratification

According to 2013 ESH/ESC global cardiovascular risk stratification [1], this patient has very high cardiovascular risk (grade 3 HTN + 1 asymptomatic organ damage).

Prescriptions

- Olmesartan 40 mg + amlodipine 5 mg (confirmed)
- Atorvastatin 20 mg (confirmed)

5.3   Follow-Up (Visit 2) After 3 Months

At follow-up visit after 12 weeks, the patient is still asymptomatic and in good clinical conditions. He reports adherence to treatment and good home values of blood pressure. No drug-related side effects are reported.

Physical Examination

- Weight: 88 kg.
- Body mass index (BMI): 29.4 kg/m^2.
- Resting pulse: regular rhythm with normal heart rate (70 beats/min).
- Mean values at home were normal. Other clinical parameters are substantially unchanged.

Blood Pressure Profile

- Home BP (average): 130/75 mmHg
- Sitting BP: 120/75 mmHg
- Standing BP: 130/70 mmHg

Current Treatment

- Olmesartan 40 mg + amlodipine 5 mg
- Atorvastatin 20 mg

Stress Test

Test performed on cycle interrupted at 150 W. No signs or symptoms of stress-induced myocardial ischaemia were recorded during exercise (Fig. 5.3).

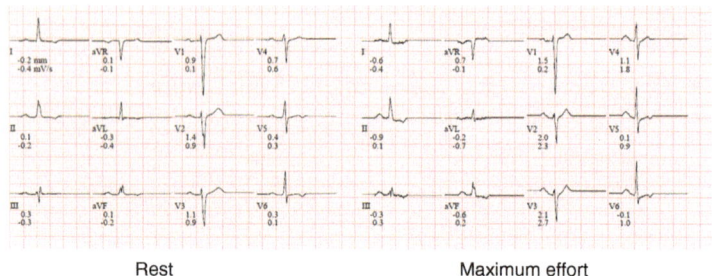

FIGURE 5.3 12-lead ECG during stress test

Haematological Profile

- Haemoglobin: 16 g/dL
- Haematocrit: 47%
- Fasting plasma glucose: 100 mg/dL
- Lipid profile: TOT-C: 174 mg/dL; LDL-C: 97.2 mg/dL; HDL-C: 53 mg/dL; TG: 119 mg/dL

Prescriptions

- Olmesartan 40 mg + amlodipine 5 mg (confirmed)
- Atorvastatin 20 mg (confirmed)

5.4   Follow-Up (Visit 3) at 1 Year

The patient presents to the hypertension clinic for a control visit.

He is asymptomatic, his lifestyle has discretely improved, and he continues to practise moderate physical activity.

Physical Examination

- Weight: 88 kg.
- Body mass index (BMI): 29.4 kg/m^2.
- Resting pulse: regular rhythm with normal heart rate (64 beats/min).
- Mean values at home were normal. Other clinical parameters are substantially unchanged.

Blood Pressure Profile

- Home BP (average): 110/70 mmHg
- Sitting BP: 124/75 mmHg (right arm); 128/76 mmHg (left arm)
- Standing BP: 129/75 mmHg at 1 min

Haematological Profile

- Haemoglobin: 15.9 g/dL
- Haematocrit: 45.5%
- Fasting plasma glucose: 98 mg/dL
- Lipid profile: TOT-C: 167 mg/dL; LDL-C: 100.8 mg/dL; HDL-C: 54 mg/dL; TG: 61 mg/dL
- Electrolytes: sodium, 137 mEq/L; potassium, 4.0 mEq/L
- Serum uric acid: 4.0 mg/dL
- Renal function: urea, 45 mg/dL; creatinine, 0.88 mg/dL; creatinine clearance (Cockroft-Gault), 122.2 mL/min; estimated glomerular filtration rate (eGFR) (MDRD), 114 mL/min/1.73 m^2
- Urine analysis (dipstick): normal
- Albuminuria: 10.2 mg/24 h
- Normal liver function tests

12-Lead ECG

Sinus rhythm with normal heart rate (62 bpm), normal atrioventricular conduction (P-R interval 204 ms), evidence of left ventricular hypertrophy (R(I) + S(III) > 2.00 mV) (Fig. 5.4).

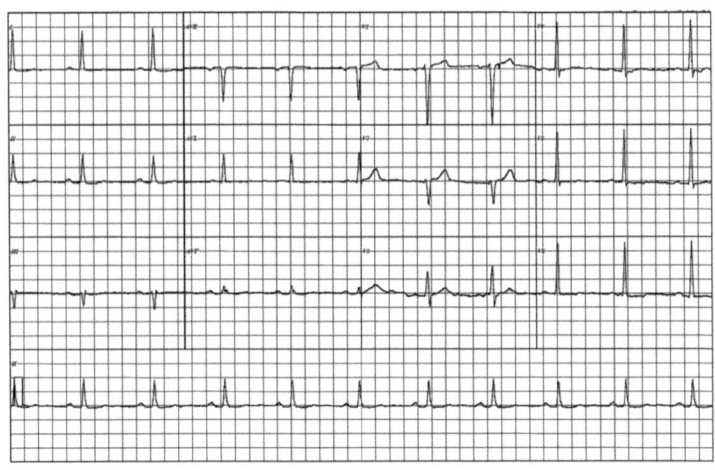

FIGURE 5.4 12-lead ECG at 1 year (follow-up visit 3)

Echocardiogram

Eccentric left ventricular hypertrophy (LV max index 57.1 g/m$^{2.7}$; relative wall thickness 0.38) with high left ventricular chamber dimension (LV end-diastolic diameter 52 mm) and volume (82.20 cm^3/m^2), normal ejection fraction (63%), dilated aortic root (42 mm), normal left atrium, absence of pathological findings on the right ventricle and pericardium.

Aortic (++) regurgitation at Doppler ultrasound examination.

Carotid Ultrasound

Both common carotids present an increase of intima-media thickness (right, 1.0 mm; left, 1.0 mm) without evidence of significant atherosclerotic plaques.

Current Treatment

- Olmesartan 40 mg + amlodipine 5 mg
- Atorvastatin 20 mg

Q2: Which is the best therapeutic option for this patient?
Possible answers are:

1. Increase amlodipine to 10 mg.
2. Stop atorvastatin.
3. Change olmesartan with ramipril.
4. No changes.

Prescriptions

No Changes

- Olmesartan 40 mg + amlodipine 5 mg (confirmed)
- Atorvastatin 20 mg (confirmed)

5.5   Discussion

This clinical case describes a patient with unknown grade III hypertension complicated by ventricular enlargement (eccentric left ventricular hypertrophy). Arterial hypertension has been associated with development and progression of cardiac organ damage, namely, left ventricular hypertrophy, which in turn is related to an increased risk of coronary events, myocardial infarction, ischaemic stroke and congestive heart failure. For these reasons, systematic assessment of left ventricular hypertrophy in all hypertensive patients has been recently reaffirmed and promoted by 2013 ESH/ESC guidelines on the clinical management of hypertension [1], in order to properly identify and treat those hypertensive patients at high cardiovascular risk.

In a recent paper we reported that the left ventricular dilatation in hypertensive patients with normal ejection fraction is associated with high cardiovascular risk [2].

The therapeutic choice for this patient was oriented on a fixed combination therapy based on the angiotensin receptor blocker olmesartan and the calcium channel blocker amlodipine. This choice is justified by the particular efficacy of the ARB olmesartan, compared with the ACE inhibitor ramipril [3], and its ability to reduce left ventricular hypertrophy [4] and to improve left ventricular function and to ameliorate the progression of cardiac remodelling [5]. The association with amlodipine is particularly recommended for its ability to reduce the peripheral resistance and consequently the aortic regurgitation.

Take-Home Messages
Arterial hypertension has been associated to the development and the progression of cardiac organ damage.

LV hypertrophy is related to an increased risk of coronary events, myocardial infarction, ischaemic stroke and congestive heart failure.

Left ventricular dilatation in hypertensive patients with normal ejection fractions is associated with high cardiovascular risk.

The fixed combination of ARBs and calcium channel blockers is able to reduce blood pressure and related target organ damage.

References

1. Mancia G, Fagard R, Narkiewicz K, Redon J, Zanchetti A, Bohm M, et al. 2013 ESH/ESC guidelines for the management of arterial hypertension: the task force for the Management of Arterial Hypertension of the European Society of Hypertension (ESH) and of the European Society of Cardiology (ESC). Eur Heart J. 2013;34(28):2159–219.

2. de Simone G, Izzo R, Aurigemma GP, De Marco M, Rozza F, Trimarco V, et al. Cardiovascular risk in relation to a new classification of hypertensive left ventricular geometric abnormalities. J Hypertens. 2015;33(4):745–54. discussion 54

3. Malacco E, Omboni S, Volpe M, Auteri A, Zanchetti A, Group ES. Antihypertensive efficacy and safety of olmesartan medoxomil and ramipril in elderly patients with mild to moderate essential hypertension: the ESPORT study. J Hypertens. 2010;28(11): 2342–50.

4. Tsutamoto T, Nishiyama K, Yamaji M, Kawahara C, Fujii M, Yamamoto T, et al. Comparison of the long-term effects of candesartan and olmesartan on plasma angiotensin II and left ventricular mass index in patients with hypertension. Hypertens Res. 2010;33(2):118–22.

5. Sukumaran V, Watanabe K, Veeraveedu PT, Thandavarayan RA, Gurusamy N, Ma M, et al. Beneficial effects of olmesartan, an angiotensin II receptor type 1 antagonist, in rats with dilated cardiomyopathy. Exp Biol Med. 2010;235(11):1338–46.

Clinical Case 6
Patient with Hypertension and Right Ventricular Enlargement

6.1 Clinical Case Presentation

A 68-year-old, Caucasian male was admitted to the outpatient clinic for recent shortness of breath. He referred having experienced increased shortness of breath and fatigue over the last 5 months and, since then, having reduced his level of physical activity. He also reports muscle pain in the calves of both legs, mostly occurring when he increases the speed of walk and disappearing with rest.

He has history of systemic sclerosis, essential hypertension, chronic obstructive pulmonary disease (COPD) and atrial fibrillation. He was diagnosed with systemic sclerosis 10 years before.

Hypertension was diagnosed 8 years before and treated with amlodipine 5 mg.

Atrial fibrillation was diagnosed approximately 2 years before, when he underwent direct current (DC) shock to restore sinus rhythm. One year before, the patient had recurrent atrial fibrillation and started to assume bisoprolol 2.5 mg daily and apixaban 2.5 mg twice daily.

COPD was diagnosed 15 years before and treated with oxygen therapy.

He reported to assume the following medications: bisoprolol 2.5 mg, apixaban 2.5 mg twice a day, amlodipine

R. Izzo, *Hypertension and Cardiac Organ Damage*,
Practical Case Studies in Hypertension Management,
DOI 10.1007/978-3-319-56080-9_6,
© Springer International Publishing AG 2017

5 mg daily, furosemide 25 mg daily, metilprednisolon 4 mg daily, tiotropium 1 puff daily, fluticasone 2 puff daily and oxygen therapy.

Family History

He has paternal history of hypertension, myocardial infarction and diabetes and maternal history of systemic lupus and stroke. He also has one sibling with hypertension and hypercholesterolaemia.

Clinical History

Former smoker (more 20 cigarettes daily) for more than 40 years, non-smoker for 1 year at presentation to the clinic. He also has one additional modifiable cardiovascular risk factor: sedentary life habits. There are no further cardiovascular risk factors, associated clinical conditions or non-cardiovascular diseases.

Physical Examination

- Weight: 65 kg.
- Height: 165 cm.
- Body mass index (BMI): 23.88 kg/m^2.
- Waist circumference: 90 cm.
- Respiration: diminished vesicular sounds.
- Heart sounds: S1–S2 is diminished. S3 is heard at the apex. A holosystolic murmur (IV/VI Levine) is heard best at the left lower sternal border. In addition, the murmur intensity increases with inspiration.
- There are mild oedema of both lower extremities and hepatojugular reflux (an increase in the JVP more than 4 cm).
- Examination of the abdomen: the anterior wall is round and soft. The liver edge is palpable. The spleen is not palpable.

- Resting pulse: irregular rhythm with a normal heart rate of 70 beats/min.
- Carotid arteries: no murmurs.
- Femoral and foot arteries: diminished peripheral pulses.

Haematological Profile

- Haemoglobin: 11.3 g/dL
- Haematocrit: 37 %
- Fasting plasma glucose: 87 mg/dL
- Lipid profile: total cholesterol (TOT-C): 128 mg/dL; low-density lipoprotein cholesterol (LDL-C): 75 mg/dL; high-density lipoprotein cholesterol (HDL-C): 44 mg/dL; triglycerides (TG): 60 mg/dL
- Electrolytes: sodium, 140 mEq/L; potassium, 4.8 mEq/L
- Serum uric acid: 6.2 mg/dL
- Renal function: urea, 49 mg/dL; creatinine, 1.17 mg/dL; estimated glomerular filtration rate (eGFR) (MDRD), 66 mL/min/1.73 m^2
- VES: 43 mm
- PCR 1.2 mg/dL
- IgA, IgG, IgM: normal
- C3: 82 (normal range 90–207)
- C4: 14.4 (normal range 17–52)
- Urine analysis (dipstick): normal
- Normal liver function tests
- Normal thyroid function tests

Blood Pressure Profile

- Home BP (average): 130/80 mmHg
- Sitting BP: 123/76 mmHg (right arm); 118/71 mmHg (left arm)
- Standing BP: 122/77 mmHg at 1 min

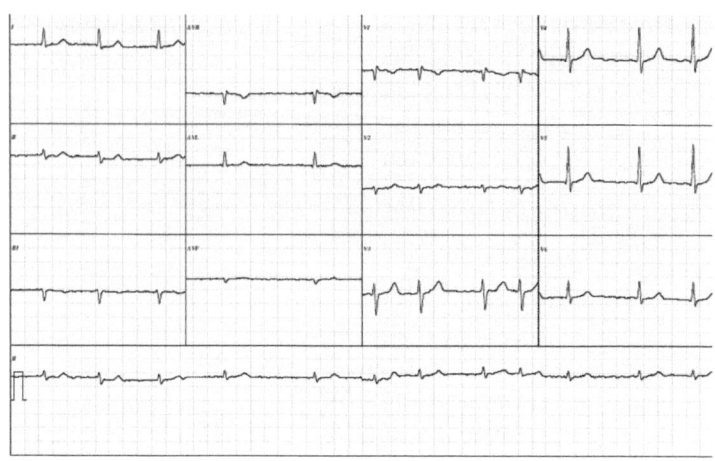

<small>FIGURE 6.1</small> 12-lead ECG at the first available visit

12-Lead ECG

Atrial fibrillation with a heart rate of 70 bpm (Fig. 6.1).

Chest X-Ray

Chest X-ray showed (Fig. 6.2):

- Abnormally large amounts of air spaces in the lung
- A flattened diaphragm
- An enlargement of the diameter of the right descending branch of the pulmonary artery (sign of pulmonary arterial hypertension — arrow)
- Paucity of vascular markings in the lung (arterial deficiency)

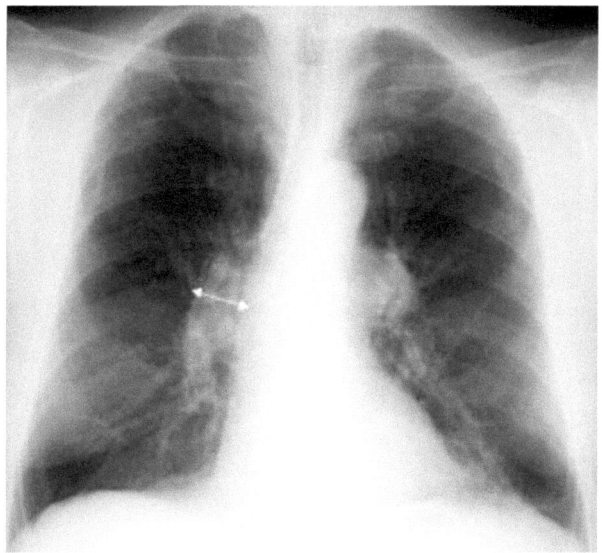

FIGURE 6.2 Chest X-ray at the first available visit

Echocardiography

The echocardiography showed severe right ventricular dilatation with global hypokinesia (TAPSE 10 mm), right atrial enlargement (RA area 3.7 cm^2), severe tricuspid regurgitation, severe pulmonary arterial hypertension (PAPs 75 mmHg; inferior vena cava 38 mm), concentric left ventricular rearrangement (LV mass indexed 45.2 g/m$^{2.7}$, relative wall thickness 0.44) with normal chamber dimension (LV end-diastolic diameter 45 mm), impaired left ventricular relaxation (E/A ratio < 1) at both conventional and tissue Doppler evaluations and normal ejection fraction (LV ejection fraction 62%) (Figs. 6.3, 6.4 and 6.5).

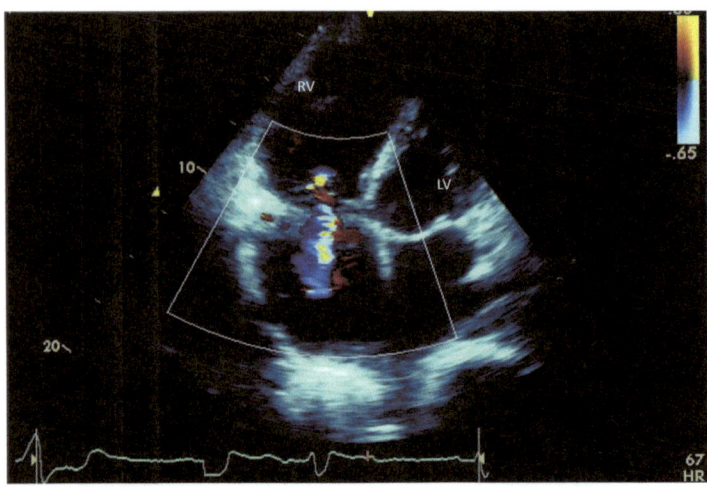

FIGURE 6.3 Echocardiography at the first visit

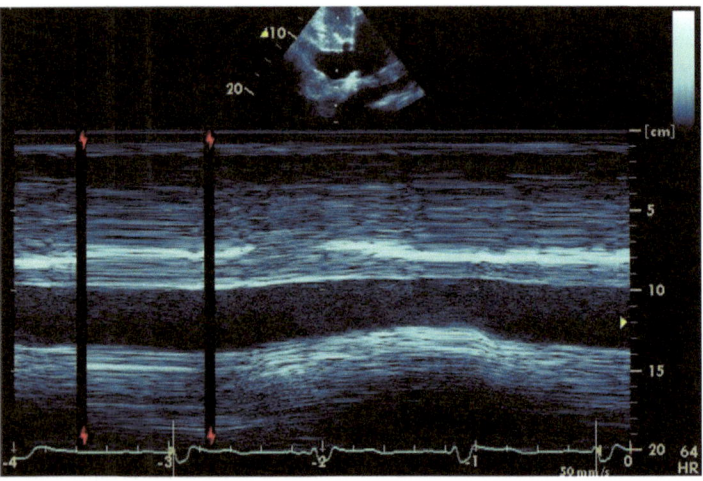

FIGURE 6.4 Inferior vena cava

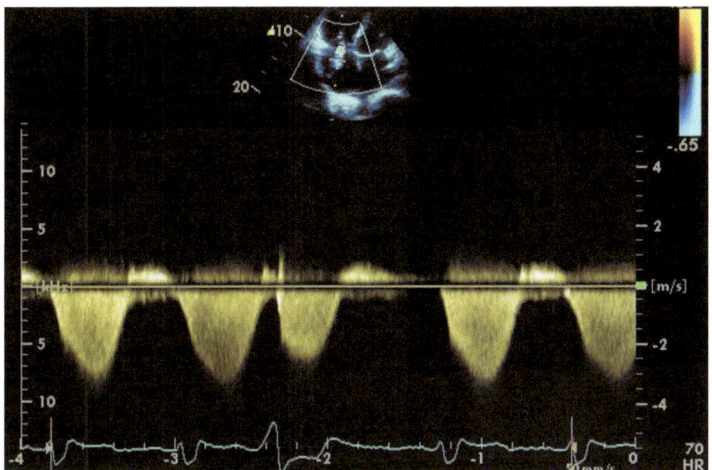

FIGURE 6.5 Tricuspid Doppler

Vascular Ultrasound

Carotid vascular ultrasound showed atherosclerotic plaques at carotid bulb (max. 1.5 mm) and the internal carotid artery (max. 1.7 mm), bilateral.

Lower Limbs

Thrombotic occlusion of the superficial femoral artery bilaterally, with deep femoral artery rehabilitation.

Diagnosis

Severe pulmonary hypertension in patient with systemic sclerosis, COPD and atrial fibrillation in patient with arterial hypertension, left ventricular hypertrophy with severe right ventricular hypokinesia, carotid plaque, thrombotic occlusion of the superficial femoral artery bilaterally.

Treatment Evaluation

- Start canrenone 25 mg three times a week.
- Indication for cardiac catheterization.

Prescriptions

- Periodical BP evaluation at home according to recommendations from guidelines
- Low-calorie and low-salt intake

6.2   Follow-Up (Visit 1) at 6 Weeks

At follow-up visit, the patient reports dyspnoea for minor efforts and asthenia. No significant changes of renal function were documented.

He also reports good adherence to prescribed medications without adverse reactions or drug-related side effects.

Physical Examination

- Weight: 65 kg.
- Resting pulse: irregular rhythm, heart rate: 67 beats/min.
- Respiration: basal fine crepitations.
- Heart sounds: a holosystolic murmur (IV/VI Levine) is heard best at the left lower sternal border.

Blood Pressure Profile

- Home BP (average): 110/70 mmHg
- Sitting BP: 120/80 mmHg (left arm)
- Standing BP: 115/85 mmHg at 1 min

12-Lead Electrocardiogram

Atrial fibrillation with a heart rate of 70 bpm.

Cardiac Catheterization

Moderate precapillary pulmonary hypertension, with a wedge pressure of 8 mmHg, mean pulmonary arterial hypertension of 40 mmHg and cardiac index of 1.94 L/min/m².

Diagnosis

Moderate precapillary pulmonary hypertension in patient with systemic sclerosis, COPD and atrial fibrillation.

Q1: Which is the best therapeutic option in this patient?
Possible answers are:

1. No changes.
2. Stop canrenone.
3. Start bosentan.
4. Stop apixaban.

Treatment Evaluation

- Start bosentan 125 mg twice a day.

6.3   Follow-Up (Visit 2) at 3 Months

At follow-up visit, the patient is in good clinical condition, having New York Health Association (NYHA) class II. No significant changes of renal function were documented.

Physical Examination

- Weight: 65 kg.
- Resting pulse: irregular rhythm with a mean heart rate of 75 beats/min.
- Respiration: diminished vesicular sounds.
- A holosystolic murmur (IV/VI Levine) is heard best at the left lower sternal border.

Blood Pressure Profile

- Home BP (average): 105/65 mmHg
- Sitting BP: 123/74 mmHg (left arm)
- Standing BP: 133/78 mmHg at 1 min

Treatment Evaluation

- Continue ongoing therapy.

Prescriptions

- Periodical BP evaluation at home according to recommendations from current guidelines.
- Periodical assessment of electrolytes and renal function.

6.4   Follow-Up (Visit 3) at 1 Year

At follow-up visit, the patient is in good clinical condition, having NYHA class II.

Physical Examination

- Weight: 64 kg.
- Resting pulse: irregular rhythm with 72 beats/min.
- Absence of peripheral oedema.

- Respiration: normal.
- Heart sounds: a holosystolic murmur (IV/VI Levine) is heard best at the left lower sternal border.

Haematological Profile

- Haemoglobin: 12.2 g/dL
- Haematocrit: 39%
- Fasting plasma glucose: 91 mg/dL
- Lipid profile: TOT-C: 137 mg/dL; LDL-C: 70 mg/dL; HDL-C: 44 mg/dL; TG: 115 mg/dL
- Electrolytes: sodium, 140 mEq/L; potassium, 4.4 mEq/L
- Serum uric acid: 5.7 mg/dL
- Renal function: urea, 54 mg/dL; creatinine, 1 mg/dL; estimated glomerular filtration rate (eGFR) (MDRD), 79 mL/min/1.73 m^2
- Urine analysis (dipstick): normal
- Normal liver function tests
- Normal thyroid function tests

Blood Pressure Profile

- Home BP (average): 110/70 mmHg
- Sitting BP: 130/80 mmHg (left arm)
- Standing BP: 128/86 mmHg at 1 min

Lead Electrocardiogram

Atrial fibrillation with an average heart rate of 70 bpm.

Echocardiography

The echocardiography showed severe right ventricular dilatation with global hypokinesia (TAPSE 12 mm), right atrial enlargement, severe tricuspid regurgitation, severe pulmonary hypertension (PAPs 65 mmHg), concentric left ventricular rearrangement (LV mass indexed 40.9 g/m$^{2.7}$, relative wall thickness 0.5) with normal chamber dimension (LV end-diastolic diameter 44 mm), impaired left ventricular relaxation (E/A ratio < 1) at both conventional and tissue Doppler evaluations and normal ejection fraction (LV ejection fraction 58%).

Current Treatment

- Bisoprolol 2.5 mg
- Apixaban 2.5 mg twice a day
- Amlodipine 5 mg daily
- Furosemide 25 mg daily
- Metilprednisolon 4 mg daily
- Tiotropium 1 puff daily
- Fluticasone 2 puffs daily
- Bosentan 125 mg twice a day
- Oxygen therapy

Q2: Which is the best therapeutic option in this patient?
Possible answers are:

1. No changes.
2. Increase bisoprolol to 5 mg.
3. Stop bosentan.
4. Stop oxygen.

Treatment Evaluation

- No change

Prescriptions

- Periodical BP evaluation at home according to recommendations from current guidelines
- Regular physical activity and low-salt intake

- Periodical control of routine chemistry
- Periodical control by immunological specialist

6.5 Discussion

This clinical case describes a patient with hypertension, COPD and systemic sclerosis. He has also atrial fibrillation, left ventricular hypertrophy with severe right ventricular hypokinesia, carotid plaque, thrombotic occlusion of the superficial femoral artery bilaterally and severe pulmonary arterial hypertension. According to the 2013 European Society of Hypertension (ESH)/European Society of Cardiology (ESC) guidelines on the clinical management of hypertension [1], this patient presents a very high cardiovascular risk (hypertension, left ventricular hypertrophy, carotid plaque and lower extremities peripheral artery disease).

Furthermore, he also has systemic sclerosis and COPD. Systemic sclerosis was frequently associated with pulmonary artery hypertension [2] and has a worse prognosis with a median survival of 3 years after diagnosis often caused by right ventricular failure [3].

In addition to antihypertensive therapy combining a calcium channel blocker (amlodipine) and a diuretic (furosemide), we prescribed bosentan 125 mg bid. Bosentan is an ET-1 receptor antagonist, able to improve the patient's functional status and other indices of pulmonary hypertension-related morbidity. It is currently clinically used for this condition [4] and is well tolerated at a dose of 125 mg twice daily [5].

Several observational studies, including the Australian Scleroderma Cohort Study, have suggested a survival benefit with anticoagulation in patients with pulmonary hypertension [6–9]. For these evidences and for contemporary presence of atrial fibrillation, we prescribed an anticoagulant in our patient.

Take-Home Messages
Systemic sclerosis is frequently associated with pulmonary artery hypertension.

When these patients have concomitant right ventricular failure, the prognosis is inauspicious.

Bosentan is an ET-1 receptor antagonist, able to improve patient's functional status and other indices of pulmonary hypertension-related morbidity.

References

1. Mancia G, Fagard R, Narkiewicz K, Redon J, Zanchetti A, Bohm M, et al. 2013 ESH/ESC guidelines for the management of arterial hypertension: the Task Force for the Management of Arterial Hypertension of the European Society of Hypertension (ESH) and of the European Society of Cardiology (ESC). Eur Heart J. 2013;34(28):2159–219.
2. Chaisson NF, Hassoun PM. Systemic sclerosis-associated pulmonary arterial hypertension. Chest. 2013;144(4):1346–56.
3. Tedford RJ, Mudd JO, Girgis RE, Mathai SC, Zaiman AL, Housten-Harris T, et al. Right ventricular dysfunction in systemic sclerosis-associated pulmonary arterial hypertension. Circ Heart Fail. 2013;6(5):953–63.
4. Budhiraja R, Tuder RM, Hassoun PM. Endothelial dysfunction in pulmonary hypertension. Circulation. 2004;109(2):159–65.
5. Rubin LJ, Badesch DB, Barst RJ, Galie N, Black CM, Keogh A, et al. Bosentan therapy for pulmonary arterial hypertension. N Engl J Med. 2002;346(12):896–903.
6. Nikpour M, Stevens W, Proudman SM, Buchbinder R, Prior D, Zochling J, et al. Should patients with systemic sclerosis-related pulmonary arterial hypertension be anticoagulated? Intern Med J. 2013;43(5):599–603.
7. Johnson SR, Mehta S, Granton JT. Anticoagulation in pulmonary arterial hypertension: a qualitative systematic review. Eur Respir J. 2006;28(5):999–1004.

8. Preston IR, Roberts KE, Miller DP, Sen GP, Selej M, Benton WW, et al. Effect of Warfarin treatment on survival of patients with pulmonary arterial hypertension (PAH) in the registry to evaluate early and long-term PAH disease management (REVEAL). Circulation. 2015;132(25):2403–11.
9. Caldeira D, Loureiro MJ, Costa J, Pinto FJ, Ferreira JJ. Oral anticoagulation for pulmonary arterial hypertension: systematic review and meta-analysis. Can J Cardiol. 2014;30(8):879–87.